80 Recipes For Beauty Face Masks

And a complete guide, to create your own combinations

More books by Evelyn Key:

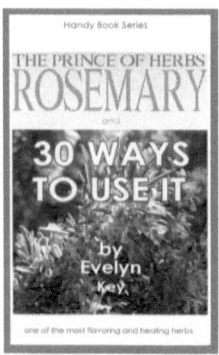
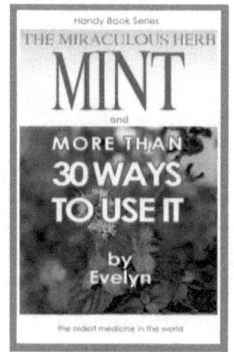

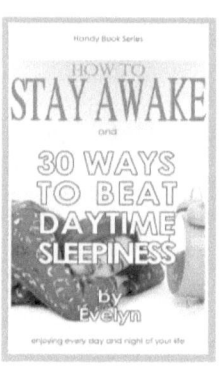
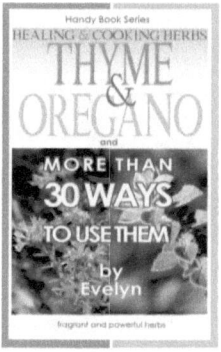

80 Recipes for Beauty Mask Recipes
And a complete guide, to create your own combinations

Evelyn Key

Handy Book Series
2014

First Printing: 2014

ISBN 978-1-312-60404-9

Evaggelia Karageorge
P.O. 1866, Agios Spyridon, Porto Rafti
Markopoulo, Attica, Greece, 19003

Handy Book Series
evelinbooks.wordpress.com
evelynbooks@gmail.com

Dedication

To all the optimist, happy and devoted people of this planet!

You create your life, you create the world!

Contents

Introduction

Hello!

This new book is dedicated to beauty care, and especially to face masks, made of absolutely natural ingredients. I tried to create a useful guide where one can find an extended list of recipes along with all the information needed to create their own.

That's right! There are uncounted potential natural ingredients, and probably, zillions of combinations that no book could ever cover all of them. Therefore, I thought that having the option to know which ingredients to combine for your own recipes, would definitely be much more convenient.

For that reason, I included two lists at the end of the book.

The first one is a list of constant skin issues and needs. Next to each skin condition, you will find catalogued the ingredients with the corresponding properties. For example:

Puffy eyes: cucumber, chamomile, avocado.

This way, one can easily find the components that meet their special needs.

Following, comes the list of the ingredients that have been used for the recipes in this book. Next to each ingredient, are noted their most valuable nutrients and benefits.

In addition, right before the recipes section, you will find a few pages with instructions and tips on masks application, skin types, usage frequency, and other useful stuff, such as natural scrubs and cleansings,.

Effortless, quick, inexpensive and most of all: natural and safe!

Natural face masks have at least two notable advantages:

A. They are so safe and natural that one could actually eat them.

B. Anyone can treat their skin just by using the content of their fridge and kitchen closets.

Seasonal fruits and vegetables are quite enough to provide you with numerous combinations. You don't have to find a watermelon in the heart of winter or buy a lettuce in July.

Obviously, I haven't used all the fruits and vegetables in the world, how could I? However, herein you will find plenty and probably some of the most common to all of us. There are no chemical ingredients in these recipes; in fact, you can actually eat some of them as a smoothie or... a salad!

Below each recipe, you will find a suggestion of how often can you use the mask:

Frequency: 1-2 times a week or up to 3-4 times a week.

This isn't mandatory; that is to say, you can apply it 3-4 times a week, but you don't <u>have to</u>. Applying more than one mask recipe during a week, is also possible. Remember though, that expecting actual results, means you have to apply the appropriate masks on a regular base.

Besides the frequency, there is one more note under each recipe, like a comment or complementary information. Some of the recipes include a precaution comment too.

Although I would suggest to read everything before you reach the recipes section, I know that many will skip it and go right to the "point". I say so because I do it sometimes too. For that reason, I often repeat again and again some lines, such as how to remove the mask; I just wanted to be sure that everyone will notice.

Nevertheless, whether you are familiar or not with the natural mask preparation, spend some time to have a quick look to all the information, just in case there are some details that you are not aware of.

So, enough with the talking! I truly hope you will find this book useful, handy and joyous!

I will be happy to hear your comments or suggestions.

Thank you!

... Evelyn Key

General Instructions and Tips

Beauty masks elevate the skin temperature and hydrate the keratin layer. They also improve the texture and the natural function of the skin.

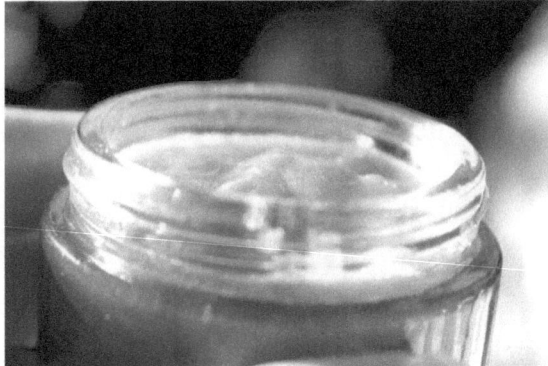

However, it is substantial to insist on totally natural ingredients, otherwise, it is almost meaningless. For example, what's the point to apply an all natural mask along with chemical creams, lotions or soaps?

So, try to keep it natural: Embrace organic and mild beauty care products.

Discover pure ways to clean and hydrate your skin.

Choose seasonal fruits and vegetables for your natural masks.

Buy organic and free of pesticides and hormones, as much as this is possible.

Apply masks when they are still fresh. Of course, storing leftovers in the fridge is reasonable, but remember that fresh is the most valuable.

Whenever is this possible, cut, chop and blend by using your hands instead of food processors, and ceramic cutlery rather than metal. Certainly, blenders provide a smoother result and this is why I often mention them in my recipes. However, it is almost a common knowledge that cutting with metal parts, destroys some of the valuable elements and therefore lowers the quality of the food.

Frequency

Even though a natural mask is pure food for the skin, there is no demand to be applied on a daily basis. The skin needs a break and also the opportunity to function by itself.

I suppose that an average of 4-5 times a week is enough.

Even so, that depends on the skin type and its particularities. In cases of a special skin condition, the mask should be applied either more often or infrequently. You will find noted instructions in each specific case.

Likewise, applying several different recipes that seem to fulfil your skin's needs, is better than to stick on a particular mask. In fact, using the same mask all the time, eventually it will lose its strength and won't have the expected effect.

Here are a few generic tips:

Exfoliating masks: best applied up to 1 time per week. Keep in mind, though, that exfoliation can be used more often on oily skins and rarely on dry skins.

Cleansing and antiseptic masks for oily skins: up to 1-2 times a week.

Moisturizing and nourishing masks: safe to use every or at least 3-4 times a week.

Soothing masks: also safe to use every day in most cases.

Tighten and firming masks: up to 1-2 times a week.

Shine masks: up to 2-3 times a week

Clay mask shouldn't be used very often: 1-3 times a month. Combined with other ingredients, clay can be adapted more frequently, like once a week. Avoid on dry skin or during skin disorders on the rise.

Masks that treat **special skin issues,** could be more beneficial applied on a regular basis, after you consult your dermatologist first.

Masks with **lemon** as an ingredient, better applied at evening or night hours; specifically, don't expose your skin directly to sunlight afterwards. Lemon is a photo-sensitiser substance and might cause some kind of skin reaction. Therefore, avoid sunbathing after applying such a mask, just to be sure and safe.

Use **shine** and **firming** masks before a date, a night out, or whenever you want to look bright.

Remember: Do not overdo with skin treatments, even if they are totally natural. Give to your skin the change to maintain its natural function.

Applying

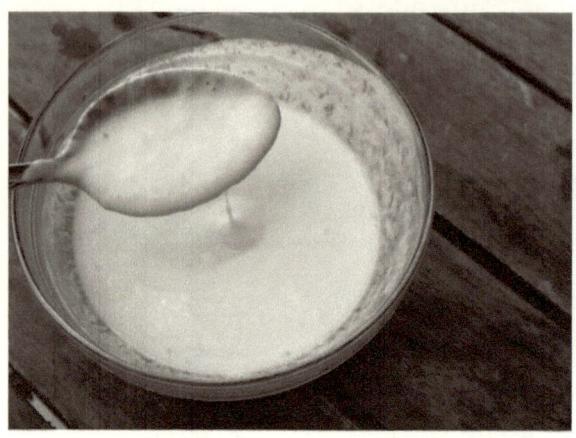

First and foremost, pick a "free of obligations" hour of the day; beauty treatment should be quality time.

- First, eliminate the risk of spilling and messing around.
- Tie up your hair, pull it back with a headband or wrap it within a towel.
- Lay a towel on the bed or seat
- Check if your accessories are clean.
- Collect the ingredients and the equipment you need for the mask preparation.
- Wash well the fruits and the vegetables.
- Clean your skin or apply a gentle peeling. In the next chapter there are noted a few ideas regarding natural skin cleansing.
- Prepare the mask.
- Apply with a cosmetics brush or with your fingertips. Try to spread a thin layer, as evenly as possible.
- Avoid the eyes and the lips, unless the mask is indicated also in those areas. Most of the masks are proper for the neck and décolleté.
- If the mixture is watery, (as many are) use a slightly damp cloth or cotton pad to apply it.
- Sit or lie down to relax. Try to avoid talking, laughing or any twitching of the facial muscles.
- Let the mask dry. However, if you feel anything unusual, like any annoyance or irritation on your skin, you better remove it.

- Remove by rinsing with plenty of water or use a wet towel, cloth or cotton pad. Make smooth movements from the forehead to the neck, without rubbing or pressing the skin.
- Initially, rinse with lukewarm water and continue with cold. The same applies if you are using a towel or cotton pad.
- Masks that contain powdery ingredients such as clay, can be removed by massaging smoothly at first, like a peeling, and then rinsing the same way as above.
- Try not to use soap to remove the mask.
- At last, apply a hydrating cream or massage with a few drops of almond or Jojoba oil, on semi wet skin because the results are better and also saves much of your hydrating product.

Skin Types

Normal is called the skin when the sebaceous glands operate in balance, and also the proportion of oil and aqueous components is right. Normal skin has fine pores and no black spots. It is soft and smooth, rarely sweats or gets greasy to the touch.

Dry skin is the one that has a reduced proportion of lipids in the hydrolipidic layer. Dry skin is matte, smooth, taut and forms wrinkles easily. No blackheads, no sweat. It is thin, rough, without elasticity.

Oily skin has an oily hydrolipidic layer because of excessive sebum secretion. Oily skin shines particularly in the T - zone. Sweats easily, and its surface is uneven, with plenty of black spots and dilated pores. It is also thick and greasy to the touch.

Finally, in cases of **Combination skin**, there is a difference of oiliness between the midline of the face and the cheeks. Combination skin has wide pores around the nose, chin and forehead, and sometimes it also has black spots.

Scrubs and Cleansing

Always apply the mask on a clean, warm and wiped skin.

Wash thoroughly the face and the neck with a gentle soap or lotion; cleaning products should be free of chemicals.

Face scrubs are also a fine cleansing solution, although they are not suitable for everyday use. Once a week is enough, depending on the skin type of course.

Rinse with warm water to open the skin pores, and help the absorption of the beneficial elements of the mask.

PEELING
Do not scrub before exfoliation or clay masks.

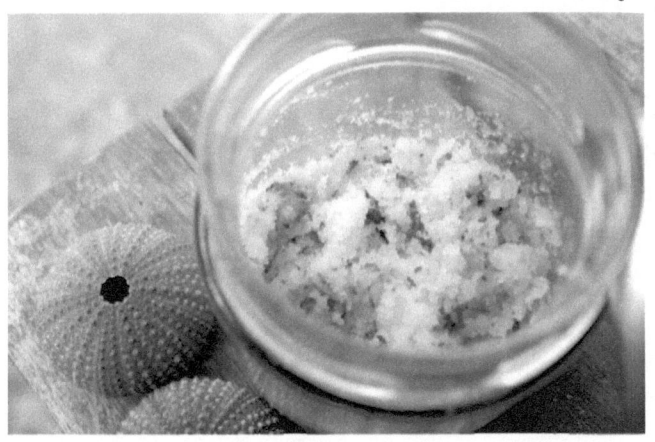

Peeling cleans your skin by removing the dead cells out of the keratin layer. It provides shine and freshness.

Face and body peeling is a valuable procedure that shouldn't be skipped. Try to apply once a week during the summer and 2 times a month in the winter.

Specifically, if your skin is:

Oily or combination skin, scrub 1-2 times a week.

Normal, scrub 1 time per week.

Dry or sensitive skin, scrub 1-2 times a month.

Caution: Avoid face scrub if you have acne or other skin disorders like eczema, wounds, etc.

Facial Scrub recipes based on skin type:
Prepare your scrubs right before use.

Normal skin:
2 tbsp brown sugar
3-2 tbsp almond or olive oil
7-8 mint leaves (optional)
How to: Crash the mint leaves with a pestle. Add the sugar and continue until they mix together. Add the oil and mix well.

Dry and Sensitive skin:
2 tbsp of oats or corn flour
Milk or olive oil
How to: Mix the flour with enough milk or olive oil to make a thick paste.

Oily skin:
1 tbsp salt
1 tbsp green clay
3 tbsp lemon juice
How to: Mix all the ingredients into a paste. If you don't have clay, use 2 tbsp of salt.

Applying the peeling:
- Tie or cover your hair with a towel.
- Put a warm wet towel on your face for two minutes.
- Apply the scrub on wet skin by rubbing gently and slowly with a cyclical movement. Use the tips of your index and middle finger.
- Work on the most troublesome areas, like the nose and the forehead.
- Apply on the neck too.
- Avoid the eye and lip areas.
- Rinse with plenty of warm water.
- Wipe gently with a towel and you are ready to apply a face mask!

CLEANSING LOTIONS
All skin types: Rose water is amazing for your skin and can be wonderfully used as a cleansing lotion.

Sensitive and dry skin: Prepare a <u>chamomile with lavender</u> infusion. When it cools, apply on your skin with a cotton pad. Rinse after 2-3 minutes with warm water, wipe gently and apply the mask.

<u>Althea root decoction</u>. Prepare, let it chill and use as above.

Oily skin: <u>1 tsp lemon with 2 tbsp milk</u>. Mix and apply the same way. Rinse with warm water, wipe gently and apply your mask.

STEAM CLEANING

In a bowl, add <u>rosemary, thyme and lavender</u> flowers (1 tbsp of each) and pour 2 cups of boiling water.

Lean your face over the steam for 5 minutes. The steam cleans the skin as it opens the pores and removes dirt. Rinse with warm water and wipe gently.

AFTER THE MASK

Always remove masks with lukewarm water, and afterwards, rinse with cold.

Tap your face and neck with a soft towel and **apply your hydrating cream**. Alternatively, **apply a light oil such as almond or Jojoba oil,** and massage gently.

Or prepare a homemade hydrating cream for all skin types:

4 tbsp bee wax

1 cup almond oil

½ cup rose water

Melt the bee wax in a double boiler (Bain Marie) and add slowly the almond oil. Remove from the heat, and add rose water while you stir until it chills. Store in a clean, sterilized jar; it doesn't need a refrigerator.

Allergies testing

Anyone can be allergic to anything without even knowing it. Even the smallest pimple can be considered as an allergic reaction.

Generally, if you don't have any allergic reactions when you eat or touch an ingredient, you are fine with it. There is though, an easy test to check any ingredients you have doubts for.

Apply on your neck at the back of your ear:

Fruits, vegetables: a small portion of flesh or a few drops of juice.

Eggs, dairy and honey: a small portion as well.

Spices and brewers yeast: a pinch dissolved in 1 tsp of water.

Essential oils and vegetable glycerine: 1 drop dissolved in 1 tsp oil (olive or almond or Jojoba, etc)

Herbs infusions, oils and apple vinegar: a few drops
.

In all cases, let it stay for 15-20 minutes and remove as you would do with the mask. If there is no skin reaction within the next 24 hours, then it is safe.

Never use essential oils directly to your skin. The same applies to vegetable glycerine. Always dissolve in other ingredients such as oils. Vegetable glycerine won't hurt your skin, but in the long term, it might dry it out.

Cautions

Be sure that you are not **allergic** to any of the ingredients you use. If you are not sure, at least test the mask in a small skin spot for before you use it. Consult your doctor for further advice.

If you are **pregnant, you** should consult your doctor before you apply anything you haven't used before during your pregnancy.

If you suffer from **acne or other serious skin disorders**, first and foremost, you should consult a specialist dermatologist who will determine the proper treatment.

If you are on **homeopathic treatment**, always check the compatibility.

Never apply masks to **wounds** or **skin disorders on the rise** unless the mask says it is specifically for that use. However, in any case of face wounds and traumas consult your doctor first.

Always consult a medical doctor about the seriousness of **skin burns**.

FACE MASK RECIPES

ACID CLEAN MASK

<u>OILY SKIN</u>, BURNS (& SUNBURNS), REDNESS.
ANTI-AGING, ANTISEPTIC, CLEANSING, REFRESHING, SKIN TEXTURE IMPROVEMENT

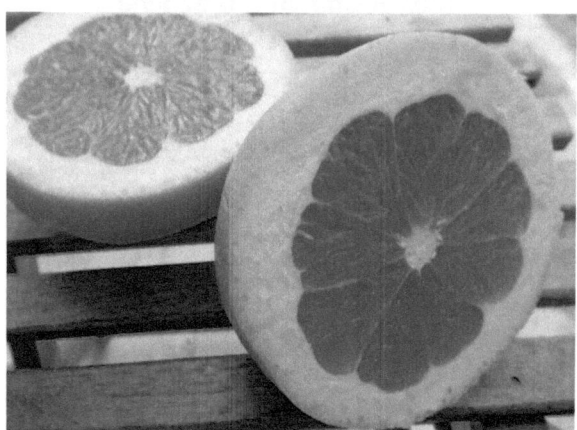

Ingredients:
1 tbsp Grapefruit juice
1 tbsp Lemon juice
2 tbsp Yogurt
How to:
In a bowl, mix the ingredients and apply the mixture on your face for 15 minutes. Remove with lukewarm water and rinse well with cold.

Note: Your skin feels lighter and cleaner.
Frequency: 1-2 times per week.

ACNE MASK-1

<u>OILY SKIN</u>, ACNE
DETOXIFYING, NOURISHING, MOISTURIZING, REFRESHING, TONIC

Ingredients:
2 tbsp Yogurt
1 tbsp fresh Tomato juice
Green Clay powder
How to:
Mix the tomato juice and the yogurt in a bowl. Add gradually the clay powder until you get a thick paste. Apply and remove with lukewarm water when it dries. Rinse with plenty cold water.

Note: This mask moisturizes, cleans deeply, detoxifies and refreshes! It also balances the skin pH.
Precaution: Do not use if acne is on the rise.
Frequency: 1 time per week at the most.

ACNE MASK-2

OILY SKIN, ACNE, IRRITATED SKIN, PIMPLES
ANTICEPTIC, EXFOLIATING, HEALING, NURISHING, RESILI-
ENCE, SOOTHING

Ingredients:
2 sprigs of Parsley
3 tbsp Yogurt
1 tsp apple vinegar

How to:
Make a parsley infusion (1 tsp parsley in 1 cup of water.) Put the yogurt into a bowl, add the apple vinegar, 1tbsp of the parsley infusion and mix. Apply the watery paste on your face for 20 minutes. Remove with lukewarm water and then rinse with cold.

Note: Don't throw away the rest of the parsley infusion. You can turn it into ice cubes for future use!

Frequency: 1-2 times a week.

ACNE MASK-3

OILY SKIN, ACNE, ECZEMA, PIMPLES, SKIN DISORDERS
ANTISEPTIC, CLEANSING, EXFOLIATING, HEALING, NOURISH-
ING, SOOTHING

Ingredients:
1 tsp Cinnamon oil
1 tbsp Yogurt
1 tsp Honey

How to:
Mix well all the ingredients to unify. Apply for about 20 minutes. Remove gently with slightly warm water and rinse well with cold.

Note: An antiseptic and detoxifying mask for deep cleansing.

Precaution: If you don't know whether you have any skin reactions with cinnamon or not, do the test: 24 hours before you apply the mask, mix a pinch of cinnamon with a small portion of yogurt. Apply on the back of the ear. Remove it after 20 minutes. If there is no reaction within the next 24 hours, then it is ok!

Frequency: 1 time per week

AFTER SUN MASK

NORMAL and DRY SKIN, ACNE, DEHYDRATED SKIN, ECZEMA, IRRITADED SKIN, REDNESS, SKIN DISORDERS

ANTI-WRINKLE, MOISTURE, REJUVENATING, SMOOTHNESS

Ingredients:

2 tbsp Mango puree

1 tsp Honey

1 tbsp Yogurt

A pinch of Turmeric

2 drops Sandalwood essential oil

How to:

Mix all the ingredients to unify. Apply on your face for 15 minutes. Rinse with lukewarm water at first and then with cold.

Note: This mask will relieve any irritation after sun bathing.

Precaution: Never use essential oils directly to your skin, but only mixed with other ingredients.

Frequency: 2-3 times a week

AFTER SUN MASK-2

ALL SKIN TYPES, SUNBURNS

FIRMING – NOURISHING – RECONSTRUCTING

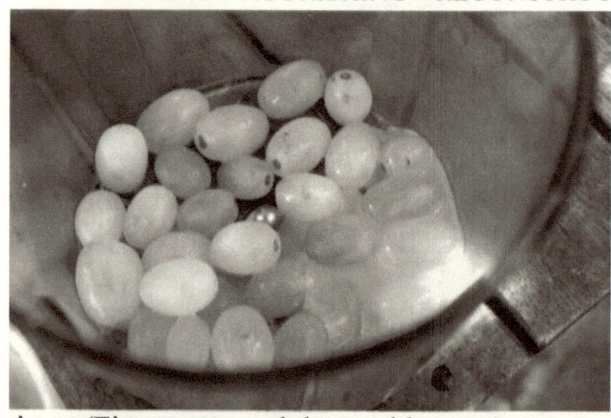

Ingredients:
1 cup green Grapes (with no seeds)
1 tbsp Honey
1 Egg yolk

How to:
Put all the ingredients in the blender and blend. Apply the mixture on your face for 15 minutes and rinse. (First warm and then cold water)

Note: This mask treats the skin after a long, summer sun exposure.

Frequency: up to 2-3 times a week.

AFTER SUN MASK-3
<u>NORMAL and DRY SKIN</u>, BURNS, INFLAMMATION
ANTI-WRINKLE, MOISTURIZING, NOURISHING, RESILIENCE, SOOTHING, PROTECTING

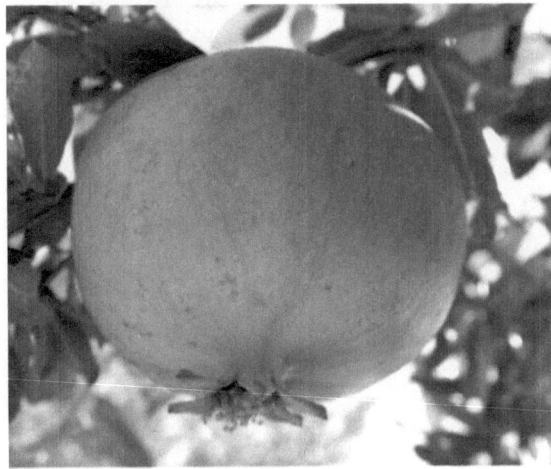

Ingredients:
½ cup Pomegranate
1 tbsp olive oil or honey
2 tbsp Yogurt
How to:
Blend all the ingredients into a paste. Apply for 20 minutes. Remove with lukewarm water and rinse with cold.
Note: Be careful with the fruits that stain, like pomegranate. Cover your clothes or furniture.
Frequency: up to 3-4 times a week

ANTI-AGING MASK-1
<u>NORMAL, DRY SKIN,</u> PREMATURE AGING
ANTI-AGING, MOISTURIZING, SKIN IMPROVEMENT
Ingredients:
½ Banana
2 tsp organic raw Cocoa
½ tsp Honey
How to:
Blend all the ingredients into a smooth paste. Add a little water (1-2tsp) if needed. Apply on your face and neck for 15 minutes. Rinse well (lukewarm-cold).
Note: A nourishing combination, especially for dry, tired and mature skins.
Frequency: up to 4-5 times a week.

ANTI-AGING MASK-2
<u>NORMAL, COMBINATION and DRY SKIN</u>, PREMATURE AGING, SKIN DISORDERS
CLEANSING, HEALING, MOISTURIZING, NOURISHING, SKIN IMPROVEMENT

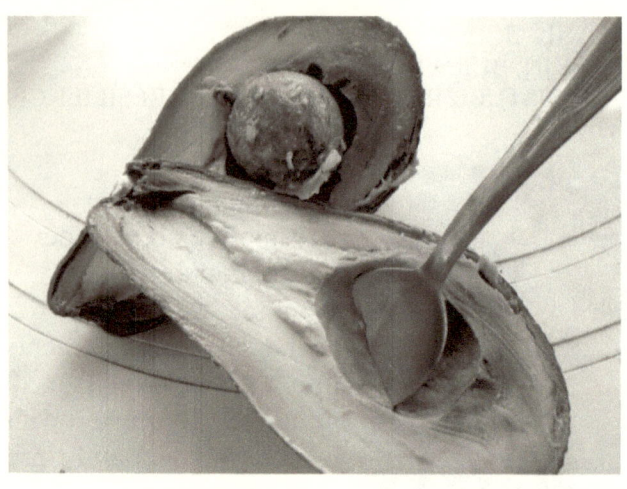

Ingredients:
1 Avocado
1 Carrot
½ cup of fresh Milk
1 Egg yolk
2 tbsp Honey
How to:
Peel the avocado and the carrot. Remove the avocado kernel and put the flesh in the blender. Boil or steam the carrot until it gets softer. Add it in the blender too, so the rest of the ingredients and blend to make a fine paste. Apply on face and neck for 15 minutes. Remove with a gentle soap (if necessary) and plenty of lukewarm water. Rinse again with cold water.

Note: This mask is good for almost any kind of skin. Nourishes and moisturizes, especially the dry skins or with issues such as colour irregularities.

Frequency: up to 3-4 times a week.

ANTI-AGING MASK-3
ALL SKIN TYPES, TIRED SKIN
ANTI-AGING, CELL REPRODUCTION, MOISTURIZING, NOURISHING, RESILIENCE, TONIC

Ingredients:
1 tsp sour cream
1 Egg yolk, beaten
1 tbsp Aloe gel
How to:
Mix all the ingredients in a bowl to unify. Apply on face and neck for 20 minutes and rinse (lukewarm first, cold afterwards).

Note: This mask is perfect if you need a rejuvenating touch. Proper for tired, mature and problematic skins, while the ingredients nourish, moisturize and help the skin reconstruction.

Frequency: up to 4-5 times a week.

ANTISEPTIC MASK
OILY SKIN, ACNE
ANTI-AGING, ANTISEPTIC, EXFOLIATING

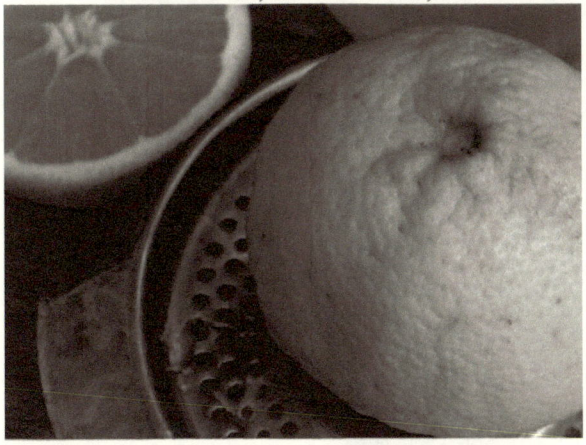

Ingredients:
1 tbsp Orange juice
1 tbsp Lemon juice
1 tbsp Grapefruit juice
5 drops of apple vinegar

How to:
Put all the ingredients in a bowl and stir well. Dip a cotton pad in the mixture and apply (except the area around the eyes.) Rinse after 15 minutes (slightly warm at first, cool afterwards).

Note: This is a liquid mask that looks more like a lotion, but it's not! You have to rinse it. If you don't have one of the ingredients, just skip it.

Frequency: 1-2 times a week.

ANTI-WRINKLE MASK
ALL SKIN TYPES
ANTI-AGING,   NOURISHING,   RECONSTRUCTIVE,   SHINE, SMOOTHING

Ingredients:
1 ripe Banana
2 tsp fresh Milk

How to:
Mash the banana, add the milk and mix into a smooth cream. Don't eat it! Apply on your face and neck for 15 minutes. Rinse with plenty of water (you know, lukewarm first, cold next).

Note: One of the easiest masks. You could try different kinds of milk, like plant milk (almond or sesame), goat, buffalo or donkey milk.

Frequency: you could do it every day, but don't. There are so many others to try.

ANTI-WRINKLE MASK-2
<u>ALL SKIN TYPES</u>
ANTI-AGING, MOISTURIZING

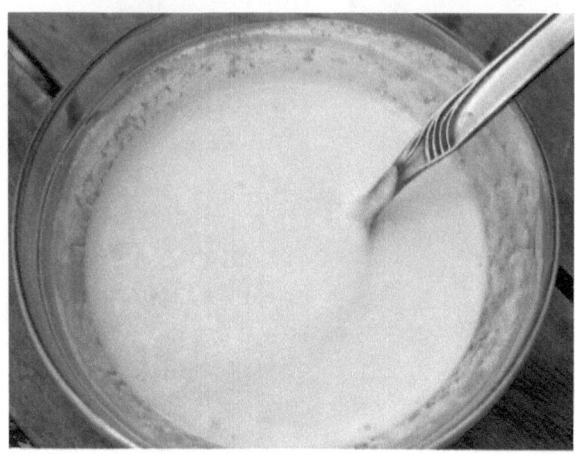

Ingredients:
2 tbsp Honey
2 tsp Milk or sour cream
How to:
Mix the honey and the milk to unify. Apply for 15 minutes. Rinse well.
Note: Sweet and simple!.
Frequency: As often as you like.

ANTI-WRINKLE MASK-3
<u>ALL SKIN TYPES</u>, DRYNESS
ANTI-AGING, ANTI-WRINKLE, CELL REPRODUCTION, SKIN IMPROVEMENT
Ingredients:
3 tbsp fresh Milk
3 tbsp Oat flour
1 tbsp mint, finely chopped
1 tbsp Spinach, finely chopped
1 tbsp Honey
How to:
Mix the milk with the flour and the honey until they unify. Add the mint and the spinach and mix well. Apply for 15-20 minutes and remove with plenty of water.

Note: Keep the leftovers of the mask in the fridge. Remember to rinse first with slightly warm water and then continue with cold.

Frequency: 1 time per week.

BRIGHT AND SMOOTH MASK
<u>ALL SKIN TYPES</u>, DRYNESS
ANTI-WRINKLE, MOISTURIZING, REFRESHING, RESILIENCE, SMOOTHING, TIGHTENING

Ingredients:
1 cup of Strawberries and raspberries or blueberries
1 cup of Yogurt
2 tbsp Honey
How to:
Wash and blend the fruits into a puree paste. In a bowl, mix the puree with the yogurt and the honey. Apply for 20 minutes and rinse.

Note: This mask is also a tasty smoothie, so enjoy the rest with a straw!

Frequency: up to 4-5 times a week.

CLEAN AND FIRM MASK-1
OILY SKIN
SHINE, TIGHTENING
Ingredients:
1 Egg white
1 tbsp Green Clay
1 tsp organic salt
How to:
Beat the egg white along with the salt. Then add the clay powder, mix well and apply immediately. When it dries, massage with your fingertips on a cyclical movement. Rinse well with slightly warm water and then with cold.

Note: This is a mask and a scrub at the same time. Removes the excess oil and cleans deeply.

Frequency: Once a week.

CLEAN AND FIRM MASK-2
NORMAL, OILY and COMBINATION SKIN
ANTI-AGING, CLEANSING, FIRMING, NURISHING, TONIC
Ingredients:
1 tbsp Green Clay
1tsp Honey
Some Milk
How to:
The milk must be at room temperature (not cold). Add the honey and stir to dissolve it. Put the clay in a small bowl, and add the

milk and honey while stirring. Mix until you get a smooth cream. Apply immediately and remove when it dries.

Note: Every time you remove a clay mask, massage gently before you rinse, for deeper cleansing.

Frequency: Once a week.

CLEAN AND FIRM MASK-3
NORMAL, OILY and COMBINATION SKIN
ANTI-AGING, CLEANSING, FIRMING, NOURISHING, SHINE

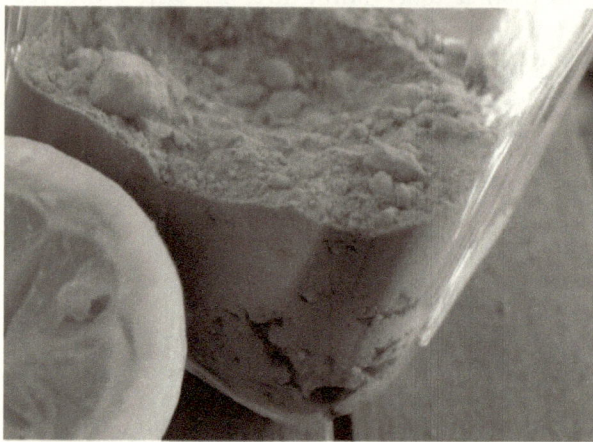

Ingredients:
1 tbsp Honey
1 tbsp Clay
1-2 tbsp sour cream
½ tsp Lemon
How to:
Mix the honey and the sour cream until the honey is dissolved. Add the lemon and pour the mixture on the clay, stirring continuously to make a paste. Apply and let it dry. Rinse well with slightly warm and cold water.

Note: Clay masks need a little more effort to remove than others. A slight massage before rinsing helps.

Frequency: Once a week.

CLEAN AND FIRM MASK-4
NORMAL, OILY SKIN
ANTI-WRINKLE, CLEANSING, TIGHTENING

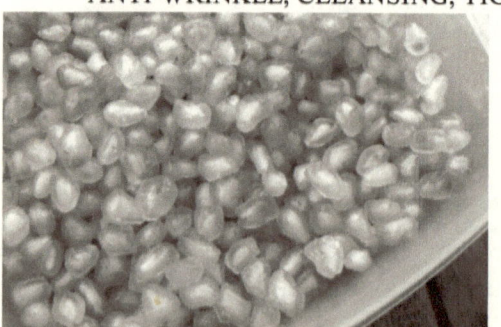

Ingredients:
1 cup of Pomegranate seeds
1 Egg white
How to:
Beat the egg white to make meringue. In a blender, blend the pomegranate seeds and then mix the two ingredients together in a bowl. Apply on

your skin for 20 minutes and rinse.

Note: You can remove the mask with lukewarm water and then use a cold natural herb lotion as the final rinse.

Frequency: up to 2 times a week.

CLEAN AND FIRM MASK-5
NORMAL and OILY SKIN
ANTI-AGING, BALLANCING, CLEANSING, NOURISHING, SOOTH-ING

Ingredients:
½ Apple
1 Egg white
2 tbsp Orange juice
1 tsp Honey
1 tsp Lemon
How to:
Mash the apple in the blender. Mix with the rest of ingredients to unify, and apply for 15 minutes. Remove with slightly warm water and rinse with cold.

Note: Face care in the heart of winter.
Frequency: 1-2 times a week.

CLEAN AND NOURISH MASK
ALL SKIN TYPES
ANTI-AGING, CLEANSING, EXFOLIATING, NOURISHING, MOIS-TURIZING

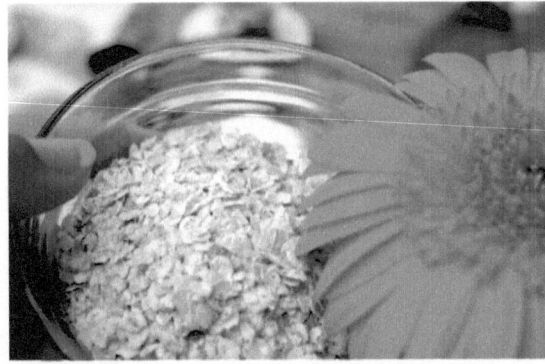

Ingredients:
2 tbsp Oats flour or flakes
2 tbsp Yogurt
1 tsp Honey
How to:
If you use oat flakes, put it in the blender and blend. In a bowl, mix the yogurt, the honey and the blended oats or flour, un-til you get a paste. Apply on your skin (face and neck) and let it for 15 minutes. Rinse. (Lukewarm/cold)

Note: This one looks good for breakfast too…! Anyway, try not to eat it all, and your skin will thank you. Remember, always apply masks to a clean face.

Frequency: up to 2-3 times a week. Dry skin: 1 time every 2 weeks.

CLEAN AND SHINE MASK
NORMAL SKIN
ANTI-AGING, CLEANSING, HEALING, NOURISHING – MOISTURIZING, PROTECTING

Ingredients:
1 cup Pomegranate seeds
2 tbsp Oat flakes
1 tbsp olive oil
1 tsp Honey

How to:
Blend all the ingredients to a fine mixture. Apply for 25 minutes and remove with slightly warm water. Rinse with cold water.

Note: This mask is also beneficial in cases of herpes virus.

Frequency: 2-3 times a week.

CLEAN AND SHINE MASK-2
NORMAL and OILY SKIN, ACNE, BURNS, INFLAMMATION, SUNBURN
ANTISEPTIC, CLEANSING, RESILIENCE, SOOTHING

Ingredients:
1 cup Pomegranate seeds
1 tbsp Yogurt
1 tbsp apple vinegar

How to:
In a blender, mash the pomegranate seeds. Mix with the other two ingredients, and apply for 10 minutes. Rinse. (Lukewarm/cold water)

Note: A proper mask for skin irritation after sunbathing. In this case you could replace apple vinegar with grape juice.

Frequency: 1-2 times a week.

DEEP CLEANSING MASK-1
OILY and COMBINATION SKIN, DULL SKIN
ANTI-AGING, CLEANSING, EXFOLIATING, NOURISHING
Ingredients:
½ medium Apple
2 tbsp Honey
1 tbsp Oat flour
How to:
Cut the apple into small pieces (don't peel), and put them in the blender. Blend 1-2 times, add the rest ingredients and blend to get a thick paste. Apply on face and neck for about 20-25 minutes and rinse well.

Note: Although I mentioned above: "for oily skins", I think that this mask is actually good for all skin types that need moisture. The deep cleansing properties make it perfect for oily skins.

Frequency: 1-2 times a week.

DEEP CLEANSING MASK-2
OILY SKIN
CLEANSING, FIRMING, NOURISHING, SHINE, TONIC
Ingredients:
1 tbsp green or white Clay
1 tsp sour cream
How to:
Mix well the ingredients into a smooth cream, adding a little more sour cream if needed. Apply the mask immediately and rinse after 20 minutes.

Note: This mask provides nourishment and smoothness while it cleans deeply.

Frequency: 1 time per week.

DEEP NOURISHING MASK
NORMAL and DRY SKIN, CRACKED SKIN, DRYNESS
ANTI-WRINKLE, CELL REPRODUCTION, NOURISHING, MOIS-TURIZING, SHINE, SKIN IMPROVEMENT
Ingredients:
2 tbsp dark chocolate powder or Cocoa
5 tbsp Honey
1 tbsp Milk

How to:

Mix all the ingredients until they unify. Apply the mixture for 20 minutes and then rinse.

Note: Always prefer organic and raw cocoa or chocolate. As for milk, you can try any milk you have available; after all, the main purpose of this book is to use the things you have in your fridge. All milks, originally, have nourishing properties. However, you can have in mind that an organic and especially a plant milk contain less toxins and additives.

Frequency: up to 4-5 times a week.

EYE MASK-1

DRY SKIN, DARK CIRCLES, DEHYDRATED SKIN, PUFFY EYES
ANTI-AGING, MOISTURIZING, NOURISHING, RECONSTRUCTION, SHINE

Ingredients:
½ ripe Avocado
½ Banana
2-3 tbsp almond oil

Preparation:

Peel and cut the fruits into the blender. Add gradually the almond oil and blend until they turn into a smooth paste. Apply the paste on the face and neck and let it for about 15-20 minutes. Remove with lukewarm water and rinse with cold.

Note: Also, proper for under the eye area, because avocado and almond oil are restorative for dark circles and puffy eyes.

Frequency: 2-3 times a week.

EYE MASK-2

ALL SKIN TYPES, DEHYDRATED SKIN, INFLAMMATION, IRRITATED SKIN, PUFFY EYES
ANTI-AGING, FRESHNESS, NOURISHING, MOISTURIZING, REFRESHING, REJUVENATING, RESILIENCE, SMOOTHNESS, TONIC

Ingredients:
2 tsp Cucumber pulp
1 tsp Yogurt

How to:

Blend the ingredients to make a smooth paste, and put it in the fridge for about 20 minutes. Then lay back, and apply the paste all around your eyes. Let it stay for 10 minutes and rinse.

Note: You can apply it on your face too. Masks with yogurt become more creamy if you put them in the fridge first.
Frequency: 2-3 times a week.

EXFOLIATE ME MASK
DRY and DULL SKIN, DRYNESS
CELL REPRODUCTION, EXFOLIATING, NOURISHING, MOISTUR-IZING
Ingredients:
2 tbsp Pumpkin puree
1 tbsp Honey
1 tbsp Yogurt
How to:
Mash the pumpkin in the blender. Mix with the other ingredients and apply for 15 minutes. Rinse well, first with lukewarm water and then cold.
Note: Use a cosmetic brush to apply the masks evenly.
Frequency: 2-3 times a week

EXFOLIATE ME MASK-2
ALL SKIN TYPES
CELL REPRODUCTION, EXFOLIATING, NOURISHING
Ingredients:
½ Apple
1 Egg yolk
1 tbsp Milk
1 tbsp Oat flakes
How to:
Put all the ingredients in the blender and blend to a smooth mixture. Apply for 20 minutes. Rinse well.
Note: Cleans and nourishes the skin!
Frequency: 1-2 times a week.

FACE LIFTING MASK-1
OILY SKIN
ANTI-AGING, SHINE, TIGHTENING, WHITENING
Ingredients:
½ Lemon juice
1 Egg white
2 tbsp Honey

How to:
Mix well the ingredients and apply on the face and neck. When it feels tightening, rinse.

Note: If it is too liquid, add one more tbsp honey.

Frequency: 2-3 times a week.

FACE-LIFTING MASK-2
NORMAL, COMBINATION and OILY SKIN
ANTI-WRINKLE, CLEANSING, FIRMING, HEALING, REJUVENATING, SHINE, TIGHTENING, WHITENING

Ingredients:
1 tbsp Honey
2 tbsp Papaya puree
½ tsp Lemon juice

How to:
Mash the papaya and mix well with the other ingredients. Apply on for 20 minutes. Rinse well. (Lukewarm/cold)

Note: Make it suitable for dry skin by replacing the lemon with an egg yolk or 1 tbsp olive oil.

Frequency: 2-3 times a week.

FACE LIFTING MASK-3
OILY and COMBINATION SKIN
COLLAGEN REPRODUCTION, FRESHNESS, MOISTURIZING, REFRESHING, RESILIENCE

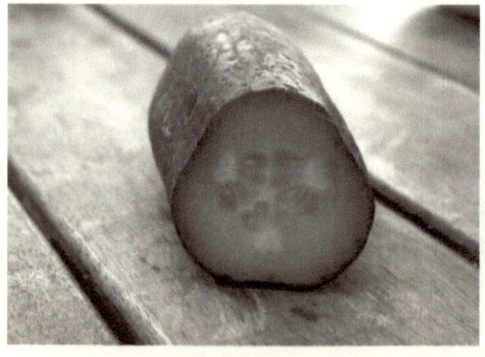

Ingredients:
½ small Cucumber
1 slice of Melon
1 Egg white

How to:
Cut the cucumber and the melon into pieces, put them in the blender and blend. Add the egg white and blend once more. Apply for 15 minutes. Rinse first with warm water and then with cold.

Note: Massage a bit the areas with the most intense problems like oiliness, acne or wide pores.

Frequency: 2-3 times a week.

FOREVER YOUNG MASK

<u>NORMAL, OILY and COMBINATION SKIN</u>
ANTI-AGING, CLEANSING, MOISTURIZING, RECONSTRUCTING

Ingredients:

1 tbsp Aloe gel

4 drops of Lemon

1 tsp Clay

1 capsule vitamin A

1 capsule vitamin E

How to:

Mix the aloe with the lemon and the vitamins. Finally, add the clay, stir well to unify and apply instantly on your face. Rinse when it dries.

Note: You can use aloe gel from the market or directly from the plant.

Frequency: 1 time per week.

HEAL AND PROTECT MASK

<u>DRY AND DISTRESSED SKIN</u>, ECZEMA, INFLAMMATION, ITCH-ING, SKIN DISORDERS
HEALING, NOURISHING

Ingredients:

2 Cabbage leaves

1 small Carrot

1tbsp Honey

3 tbsp rose water

1 tbsp brewer's yeast

How to:

Dissolve the brewer's yeast in the rose water. Wash the cabbage leaves, peel and cut the carrot and put them both in the blender. Add the yeast mixture and blend. Pour the mixture in a bowl, add the honey and mix well. Apply on your skin for 20 minutes. Rinse well.

Note: This mask can protect and refresh your skin during the winter low temperatures. Especially if you suffer from skin disorders like acne, eczema, rashes, psoriasis.

Frequency: up to 5 times a week.

HEAL ME MASK
SKIN DISORDERS
CLEANSING, HEALING, NOURISHING
Ingredients:
1 tbsp Cinnamon
2 tbsp Honey
How to:
Mix and apply on the distressed areas.

Note: whether you use it as a mask or you eat it, honey with cinnamon are a powerful combination with superb benefits for health! In cases of acne: Apply on the pimples before you go to bed. The next morning rinse with warm water.

Precaution: Try the allergy test for cinnamon: 24 hours before, mix a pinch of cinnamon with a small portion of honey, and apply it on your neck, at the back of the ear. Remove it after 20 minutes and check if any reaction appears within the next hours.

Frequency: Daily use for two weeks, removes the pimples from the root.

HEALING MASK
OILY and COMBINATION SKIN, SKIN DISORDERS
CLEANSING, HEALING, NOURISHING, SMOOTHING
Ingredients:
1 tbsp Green Clay
1 tbsp brewer's yeast
1 tsp Honey
1 tsp Orange juice
1 tsp Lemon juice
1 tbsp Calendula oil
2 drops Sandalwood essential oil
How to:
Put the lemon, the orange juice and the yeast in a small bowl and mix well. Add the honey, the Calendula oil and the sandalwood essential oil and mix again. Finally, add the clay, mix and apply on your face. Remove after 15 minutes with warm water and then rinse with cold.

Note: All the ingredients of this mask have healing properties, highly beneficial for distressed skins.

Frequency: 1-2 times a week.

HEALING CATAPLASM MASK
<u>DISTRESSED or WOUNDED SKIN</u>, ECZEMA, INFLAMMATIONS, ITCHING
RECONSTRUCTING, SOOTHING
Ingredients:
1 medium Cabbage leaf
1 tbsp almond oil
How to:
Blend the cabbage into a pulp, mix with the almond oil, and apply to the suffering skin for 15 minutes. Remove gently with a wet soft cloth or a cotton pad.

Note: This healing cataplasm should be repeated regularly until the disorder is relieved. It would be best to avoid the blender and mash the cabbage with a pestle; this way it preserves fully its healing action.

Frequency: As often as you like.

LIFT AND SHINE MASK
<u>NORMAL, OILY and COMBINATION SKINS</u>
ANTI-AGING, BALANCING, FIRMING, NOURISHING, RESILIENCE, SHINE
Ingredients:
1 Egg white
1tbsp Lemon juice
1 tsp almond oil
1 tbsp Apple puree
How to:
Mix all the ingredients together. Apply for 15 minutes and rinse.

Note: Natural masks should be applied on a regular base in order to achieve visible results.

Frequency: 1-2 time per week.

MATURE MASK
<u>DEHYDRATED and DISTRESSED SKIN</u>
ANTI-AGING, COLLAGEN PRODUCTION, HEALING, SKIN IMPROVEMENT, SOOTHING
Ingredients:
1 medium Potato

8-10 Parsley leaves
1 tbsp olive oil
1 tbsp Milk
How to:
Peel the potato and steam it. Put it in the blender, add the rest ingredients and blend. Apply on the face and neck for 20 minutes. Rinse with lukewarm water and next with cold.

Note: Try not to eat this delicious potato salad! If you are sure that the potato is free of pesticides, steam and mash it with the peel.

Frequency: up to 4-5 times a week.

MOISTURISING MASK-1
NORMAL, DRY and DESTRESSED SKIN, IRRITATED SKIN, RED-NESS, SUNBURN
ANTI-AGING, CELL PRODUCTION, COLLAGEN PRODUCTION, HEALING, MOISTURISING, RESILIENCE, SOOTHING
Ingredients:
2 tbsp Honey
1 tbsp Yogurt
2 tbsp Aloe gel
1 tsp rose water
How to:
Put the ingredients in a bowl and mix well until you get a smooth paste. Apply on the face and neck for 15-20 minutes and then rinse.

Note: Suitable for acne scars and marks or broken blood vessels.

Frequency: up to 4-5 times a week.

MOISTURIZING MASK-2
NORMAL, DRY and DISTRESSED SKIN, DRYNESS
ANTI-AGING, CLEANSING, HEALING, NOURISHING, MOISTURIZ-ING, RECONSTRUCTING
Ingredients:
½ ripe Avocado flesh
1 tbsp Tomato juice
1 tbsp Honey
How to:

Put all the ingredients in the blender and blend to a smooth paste. Apply for 20 minutes. Remove with slightly warm water and rinse well with cold.

Note: You can add some olive oil or replace the honey with it. This mask is good for delicate or dehydrated skins.

Frequency: 3-4 times a week.

NECK MASK
ALL SKIN TYPES
ANTI-WRINKLE

Ingredients:
The peels of a medium cucumber

How to:
Cover your neck skin with the peels. Wrap a towel or a scarf around your neck to hold them in place, and let for 60-90 minutes.

Note: Perfect for neck wrinkles.

Frequency: as often as you like.

NOURISHING MASK-1
NORMAL and DRY SKIN, DRYNESS
ANTI-WRINKLE, RESILIENCE, SOOTHING, NOURISHING, MOISTURIZING

Ingredients:
1 ripe Banana
1 tbsp olive oil

How to:
Mash the banana. Add the oil and mix well. Apply and rinse after 20 minutes.

Note: An 'easy to prepare' mask, perfect for tender nourishment.

Frequency: as often as you like.

NOURISHING MASK-2
DRY SKIN
ANTIAGING, CLEANSING, DETOXIFICATION, NOURISHING, MOISTURISING, SHINE

Ingredients:
3 tbsp pumpkin seeds
2 tbsp almond or olive oil

How to:

Blend the pumpkin seeds into powder. Mix well with the oil and apply on your skin for 15-20 minutes. Remove with lukewarm water and then rinse with cold.

Note: Add the oil gradually, trying not to make it too liquid.

Frequency: as often as you like.

NOURISHING MASK-3
DRY and DESTRESSED SKIN
ANTI-AGING, HEALING, NOURISHING, MOISTURIZING
Ingredients:
1 tbsp Honey
½ avocado flesh
1 Egg yolk
1 capsule vitamin E
How to:
Put the avocado in the blender and blend once. Add the egg yolk, the honey and blend to make a smooth paste. When the mixture is ready, pour into a bowl, add the vitamin E and stir. Apply and rinse after 15 minutes.

Note: A deep nourishing and moisturizing mask, very beneficial for dry skins.

Frequency: up 3-4 times a week

NOURISHING MASK-4
NORMAL and DRY SKIN
ANTI-AGING, NOURISHING, MOISTURIZING, SKIN IMPROVE-
MENT
Ingredients:
1 tbsp Honey
1 tsp Milk
1 tsp olive oil
How to:
Mix all the ingredients and apply for 20 minutes. Rinse well the usual way.

Note: Excellent for dry and tired skin.

Frequency: as often as you like.

PEEL ME GENTLY MASK
NORMAL, COMBINATION and DRY SKIN
ANTI-AGING, CLEANSING, EXFOLIATING

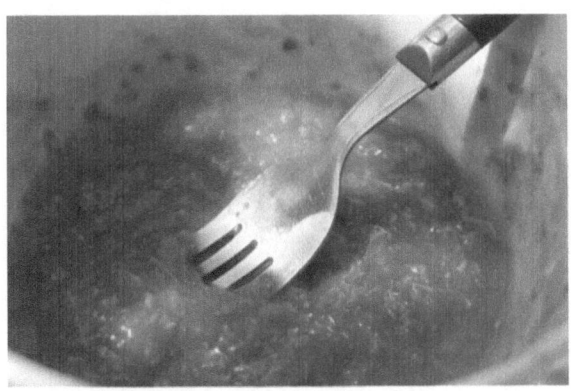

Ingredients:
2 small figs or 1 big
1 tbsp olive oil
How to:
Peel the figs, mash them in the blender and mix with the olive oil. Apply on the face and neck for 20 minutes and then rinse first with lukewarm and cold water.

Note: You can mash the figs with a fork, but a blender gives a smoother result.

Frequency: up to 3-4 times a week.

POPEYE'S MASK
ALL SKIN TYPES
ANTI-AGING, ANTISEPTIC, CLEANSING, MOISTURIZING, SHINE
Ingredients:
5 small Spinach leaves
1 tbsp Honey
1 tbsp almond oil
1 tsp Lemon juice
How to:
In a blender, blend the spinach leaves with 1-2 tsp water. Mix all the ingredients in a bowl and apply on the face for 20 minutes. Remove with slightly warm water and then rinse with cold.

Note: Take advantage of the antioxidant spinach and give your skin a winter treat.

Frequency: up to 2-3 times a week.

RECONSTRUCTING MASK
ALL SKIN TYPES, ACNE, ECZEMA, INFLAMMATION, REDNESS
ANTI-AGING, SHINE, SMOOTHING
Ingredients:
1 tbsp yeast powder
Rose water
How to:

Mix the brewer's yeast with rose water, just enough to make a paste. Apply on the face for 20 minutes (or until it dries). Afterwards, scrub gently to remove it. Rinse well (lukewarm/cold.)

Note: The brewer's yeast can be also in wet form. This mask is good for skin eczema too.

Frequency: 1-2 times a week.

Caution: Always consult your dermatologist in cases of serious skin conditions.

RECONSRUCTING MASK-2
NORMAL, DRY and COMBINATION SKIN, REDNESS
ANTI-WRINKLE, COLLAGEN PRODUCTION, EXFOLIATION, RESILIENCE
Ingredients:
1 Egg yolk
1 tbsp Kiwi puree
1 tbsp olive oil
How to:
Choose a ripe kiwi, peel it, cut into small pieces and mash them with a fork; better not use a blender. Mix with the other ingredients to unify, and apply on your face for 15 minutes. Rinse.

Note: Kiwi seeds exfoliate gently the skin. This is a quite nourishing fruit, suitable for almost all skin types.

Frequency: up to 2-3 times a week.

REFRESHING MASK
ALL SKIN TYPES, BURNS, IRRITATED SKIN, REDNESS, SUNBURN
FRESHNESS, MOISTURIZING, RESILIENCE, SOOTHING
Ingredients:
1 tbsp Watermelon
1 tbsp Cucumber
2 tbsp Yogurt
How to:
Grate the watermelon and the cucumber. Put all the ingredients in a bowl and mix. Apply on the face and neck for 20 minutes. Rinse well.

Note: This mask is very soothing for irritated skin. Better use a cosmetics brush to apply, as you should do with all the watery masks. Keep leftovers in the fridge for 1-2 days.

Frequency: as often as you like.

SENSITIVE MASK
DRY and SENSITIVE SKIN, IRRITATED SKIN, SENSITIVE SKIN
ANTI-AGING, ANTISEPTIC, MOISTURIZING

Ingredients:

2 green tea bags

1 tbsp Honey

1tsp Tomato juice

How to:

Use ½ cup of water and 2 tea bags to make the tea. Let it stand and chill for about ½ hour. Then remove the tea bags, add the honey and the tomato juice and stir well. Apply with a cosmetics brush or a cotton pad. Leave it for about 15 minutes and then rinse with luke-warm and cold water.

Note: Store the rest in the fridge for a few days.

Frequency: 1-2 times a week.

SHINE MASK-1
NORMAL, DRY and CRACKED SKIN, DEHYDRATED SKIN
CELL REPRODUCTION, DETOXIFICATION, MOISTURIZING, NOURISHING, SHINE, SKIN IMPROVEMENT

Ingredients:

3 tbsp grated dark chocolate

1 tbsp almond oil

How to:

Melt the grated chocolate in a glass or ceramic bowl over boiling water; the "bain marie" method. When the chocolate melts, add the almond oil and remove from the heat source. Stir to unify. Let it cool for a while; test it to see if you can stand it on your skin, and apply for 20 minutes. Rinse well and shine!

Note: Smooth and delicious! A mask that makes you feel as if you were in your private spa. You can use white chocolate too, but it doesn't have the antioxidant elements of the dark.

Frequency: as often as you like.

SHINE MASK-2
<u>NORMAL, OILY and COMBINATION SKINS</u>
FIRMING, TIGHTENING, MOISTURIZING

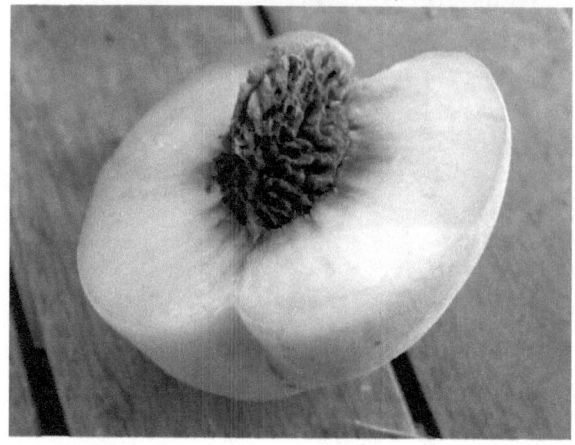

Ingredients:
1 Peach
1Egg white
How to:
Wash the peach, cut in-to pieces and put in a blender. Add the egg white and blend until it becomes a smooth cream. Apply on the face for 20 minutes and rinse well (luke-warm/cold water.)

Note: The skin feels skin tighten and moisturized. Eating peaches or drinking fresh peach juice, also helps the skin from within.

Frequency: 2-3 times a week.

SKIN DISORDERS MASK-1
<u>OILY and DISTRESSED SKIN</u>
ANTISEPTIC, CLEANSING, SHINE
Ingredients:
1 Chamomile bag
2 tbsp green Clay powder
1 tsp Lemon juice
How to:
Prepare a chamomile infusion. Put the clay in a bowl and add tablespoons of the chamomile infusion, gradually while stirring, until you get a smooth paste. Add the lemon and stir again. Apply on the face and let it until it dries. Scrub gently and rinse with plenty of wa-ter.

Note: Don't scrub if you use this mask for skin conditions such as sunburns, bunions, psoriasis, freckles etc; just rinse.

Frequency: 1 time per week.

SKIN DISORDERS MASK-2
ACNE, SPOTS and DILATED PORES
ANTI-AGING, CLEANSING
Ingredients:
1 ripe Tomato
5 drops of Lemon juice
1 tbsp Honey
How to:
Wash the tomato and put it with the other ingredients in the blender. Apply the mixture on your face and neck for 15-20 minutes. Rinse.

Note: Store the rest in the fridge for a few days. If you have wide pores, add more lemon; if you have brown spots add more honey.

Frequency: up to 3-4 times a week.

SHOOTH AND SHINE MASK
ALL SKIN TYPES, BURNS
ANTI-AGING, REFRESHING, RESILENCE, MOISTURIZING, NOURISHING, TONIC, SMOOTHING
Ingredients:
½ ripe Banana
½ small Cucumber
1 tbsp Yogurt
½ tsp Lemon juice
How to:
Mash the banana and grate the cucumber. Put the mixture in a bowl and mix with the yogurt and the lemon. Stir until they unify. Apply for 15 minutes and rinse well.

Note: A quite nourishing mask to lift up your face.
Frequency: up to -5 times a week.

SMOOTH AND SHINE MASK
ALL SKIN TYPES, PREMATURE AGING
ANTI-AGING, ANTI-WRINKLE, CLEANSING, EXFOLIATING, MOISTURIZING, SHINE, SMOOTHING
Ingredients:
1 cup of cranberries
1 tbsp Honey

1 tbsp Yogurt
1 tbsp almond butter
How to:
Put the cranberries in a blender and blend; add a little water if needed. In a bowl, mix all the ingredients into a smooth paste. Apply for 20 minutes and rinse well.

Note: You can buy almond butter from the market or prepare your own: Soak a few almonds overnight. In the morning, remove the brown peel, and put them in the blender, add water to cover and blend them well. Strain the liquid with a cheese cloth. Drink the almond milk, and use the leftovers in the cheesecloth, as almond butter.

Frequency: up to 3-4 times a week.

SMOOTH EXFOLIATE MASK
<u>DRY SKIN</u>, BLACKHEADS, BURNS, IRRITADED SKIN, SUNBURN
EXFOLIATING
Ingredients:
2 tbsp baking soda
Olive oil or Calendula oil
How to:
Mix the baking soda with olive oil (or Calendula) until you get a thick paste. Apply on the skin for 15 minutes. Rub your face, very gently, before you rinse with plenty of water.

Precaution: Do not apply to open burn wounds. If the burn or sunburn is serious (as second or third degree), you need definitely professional medical care.

Note: This mask is very beneficial for sunburns or insect bites.
Frequency: up to 2 times per month.

SOOTHING EXFOLIATE MASK
<u>DRY AND NORMAL SKIN,</u> DRYNESS, DULL SKIN
ANTI-AGING, CLEANSING, EXFOLIATING, NOURISHING
Ingredients:
1 medium Fig (peeled)
2 tbsp Pumpkin puree
1 tbsp Aloe gel
1 tsp almond oil
How to:

Cut the fig and the pumpkin into small pieces and mash them. Mix with the other ingredients to unify, and apply on the face for 20 minutes. Rinse gently.

Note: If you don't have any figs available, use 2 tbsp of apple puree instead.

Frequency: up to 3 times a week.

SOOTHING MASK
ALL SKIN TYPES, COLOR IRREGULARITIES
NOURISHING, REJUVENATE, SKIN IMPROVEMENT, SOOTHING
Ingredients:
10 leaves of fresh Mint
A pinch of Turmeric powder
1 tbsp Yogurt
How to:
Mash the mint with a pestle. Add the yogurt and mix well. Add the turmeric powder and stir to create a paste. Apply for 15 minutes and rinse.

Note: Try this mask if your skin is irritated or itching. Turmeric helps also in skin discoloration issues. Generally, this mask is suitable for several skin disorders.

Frequency: up to 2-3 times a week.

SOOTHING MASK-2
ALL SKIN TYPES, ACNE, BURNS, IRRITATED SKIN
NOURISHING, MOISTURIZING, SOOTHING
Ingredients:
1 tbsp Yogurt
1 tbsp Honey
How to:
Mix well to unify. Apply on the skin and rinse after 20 minutes (Lukewarm/cold.)

Note: This mask is perfect after sunbathing. FOR DRY SKIN: add 1 more tbsp honey. FOR OILY SKIN: add a few drops of lime.

Frequency: as often as you like.

SOOTHING MASK-3
DRY SKIN, BURNS, IRRITATED SKIN
CLEANSING, MOISTURIZING, NOURISHING, SOOTHING
Ingredients:
1 tbsp Yogurt
1 tbsp Honey
1 tsp baking soda
How to:
Mix well the yogurt with the baking soda. Add the honey and mix again. Apply for 20 minutes. Rinse.

Precaution: Do not apply to open burn wounds. If the burn or sunburn is serious (as second or third degree), you need definitely professional medical care.

Note: Instead of yogurt you can use milk or sour cream, but the result will be more watery.

Frequency: 1 time per week.

SPIDER VEINS MASK
DISTRESSED SKIN, BROKEN BLOOD VESSELS, SUNBURN
ANTI-AGING, CLEANSING, SKIN IMPROVEMENT
Ingredients:
3-4 Lettuce leaves (small to medium)
2 tbsp olive oil
½ Lemon juice
How to:
Put the lettuce leaves in a blender, add the oil and the lemon and blend. Apply for 20 minutes. Remove with a cotton pad, dipped in milk.

Note: Optionally, you can add some royal jelly to the mix (portion as a small bean.) If you have spider veins, you can use lettuce juice as a lotion morning and night. Let it dry and rinse.

Frequency: 1-2 times a week.

SUN AND YOUTH MASK
ALL SKIN TYPES, SUNBURN
ANTI-AGING, CLEANSING
Ingredients:
1 tsp Aloe gel
1 tbsp Peach puree

3 drops of Lemon.

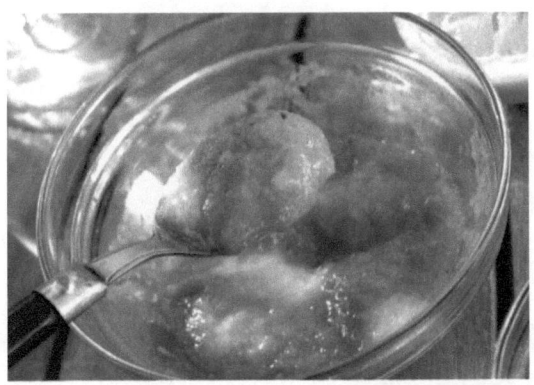

How to:
Blend half a peach to make a puree. In a small bowl, put the above ingredients and mix well. Apply on your face for 20 minutes and rinse well as usual, first slightly warm water and then cold.

Note: A pure summer recipe, perfect for after sun care! Remember eating fruits like peach is the perfect and natural sun protection!

Frequency: 3-4 times a week.

SUNBURN MASK

ALL SKIN TYPES, ACNE, BURNS, IRRITATED SKIN, REDNESS
ANTI-WRINKLE, COLLAGEN REPRODUCTION, FRESHNESS, –
RESILIENCE - SOOTHING – SUNBURN – TIRED SKIN

Ingredients:
1 tsp Aloe gel
1 tbsp Yogurt

How to:
Mix and apply for 20 minutes. Rinse well.

Note: It can't be more cool or smoother!

Frequency: Repeat 3 times a day until your sunburn resolves.

SUNBURN MASK-2

NORMAL, DRY and COMBINATION SKINS, DRYNESS, SUNBURN
ANTI-AGING, FIRMING, NOURISHING, MOISTURIZING, RESILI-
ENCE

Ingredients:
1 cup of Grape
1 tbsp olive oil
2 tbsp Yogurt
1 tbsp Honey

How to:

Mash the grapes in a blender machine. In a bowl, mix all the ingredients into a paste. Apply on your skin for 25 minutes, or longer, and rinse (Lukewarm/cold water).

Note: Whether you have a sunburn or not, you will love the touch of this nourishing and soothing mask!

Frequency: up to 4-5 times a week.

SUNSHINE MASK
NORMAL, OILY and COMBINATION SKIN
CLEANSING, NOURISHING, SUN PROTECTION

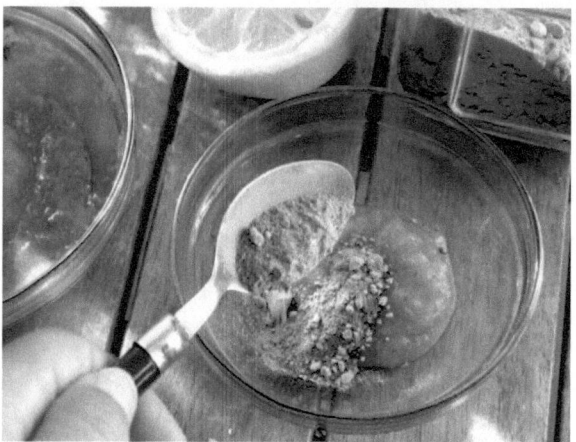

Ingredients:
1 tbsp Peach puree
1 tbsp green tea
1 tsp Clay powder
How to:
Make a green tea infusion; since you're going to use only 1 tbsp, drink the rest. In a small bowl, put all the ingredients and stir to mix well. Apply instantly. Rinse after 15-20 minutes.

Note: If you don't want to drink the rest of the tea, make some ice cubes with it, and use them any time you want to refresh your face skin.

Frequency: 1 time per week.

SWEET CLEANING
ALL SKIN TYPES
ANTI-AGING, COLLAGEN REPRODUCTION, HEALING, SKIN IMPROVEMENT

Ingredients:
2 tbsp sweet potato puree
1 tbsp Honey
How to:
Boil the sweet potato and mash it. In a bowl, put the ingredients and mix. Apply on your face for 25 minutes and rinse.

Note: Add a few drops of lemon if your skin is oily. Don't throw away the water from the potato. Keep it in the fridge and use it as a tonic and soothing lotion.

Frequency: as often as you like.

TIGHTENING MASK
NORMAL and DRY SKIN
FIRMING, MOISTURIZING, SMOOTHING
Ingredients:
1 Egg white
1tbp Honey
2 tbsp flour (optionally Oat flour)
1 tsp vegetable glycerine
How to:
In a bowl, mix the egg white, the glycerine and the honey until they unify. Add the flour and mix again until you get a thick batter. Apply on the face and neck for 10-15 minutes. Remove with slightly warm water and then rinse with cold.

Note: Massage gently while you remove, to make a slight peeling.

Frequency: 1 time per week.

TONIC MASK-1
ALL SKIN TYPES, DULL & TIRED SKIN
NOURISHING, TONIC
Ingredients:
1 Egg yolk
1 tbsp Honey
1 drop of Mint essential oil
How to:
Mix well the ingredients and apply on the face. Rinse after 15 minutes.

Note: This mask relieves pain and itching of sick or tired skin.
Frequency: 2-3 times a week.

TONIC MASK-2
NORMAL, OILY and COMBINATION SKIN
ANTI-AGING, CLEANSING, TONIC
Ingredients:

1 small Cucumber
1 Egg white
1 tsp Lemon juice
How to:
Grate the cucumber. In a bowl, add the egg white, the lemon and mix well. Add the grated cucumber and mix. Apply for 15 minutes and rinse well.

Note: Better avoid sun exposure after applying masks with lemon, because it is a photo-sensitising substance and might cause skin reactions.

Frequency: up to 2 times a week.

TONIC MASK-3
ALL SKIN TYPES
ANTI-WRINKLE, HEALING, NOURISHING, REJUVENATING, SKIN IMPROVEMENT, TONIC
Ingredients:
½ Cucumber
½ tsp Turmeric
1 tbsp sour cream
1 capsule vitamin A
How to:
Grate the cucumber. In a bowl, mix well all the ingredients and apply for 15 minutes. Rinse.

Note: Place slices of cucumber on your eyes while relaxing.

Frequency: 3-4 times a week.

TROUBLED SKIN MASK-1
ALL SKIN TYPES, BURNS
NOURISHING, MOISTURE
Ingredients:
1 tbsp Honey
1 tbsp Yogurt
1 tbsp Lemon juice
How to:
Mix well all the ingredients to unify. Apply on the skin and let it for 15 minutes before you rinse (lukewarm/cold.)

Note: A nourishing mask for all skin types, especially those that need a soothing touch.

Frequency: 2-3 times a week.

TROUBLED SKIN MASK-2
DRY and COMBINATION SKIN
ANTI-AGING, CLEANSING, EXFOLIATING, NOURISHING, MOIS-TURIZING, REFRESHING, RESILIENCE, SMOOTHING
Ingredients:
1 medium Cucumber
1 cup Oat flakes
2 tbsp Yogurt
How to:
Put the oat flakes in the blender and blend. Add the cucumber and blend again. Pour the mixture in a bowl, add the yogurt and mix to get a paste. Apply on your skin for 30 minutes and rinse well as usual.
Note: This mask is suitable for irritated skin that needs to be refreshed and moisturized.
Frequency: 2-3 times a week.

WHITENING MASK-1
NORMAL and OILY SKINS
ANTI-AGING, FIRMING, SHINE, SKIN IMPROVEMENT, TIGHTEN-ING, TONIC, WHITENING
Ingredients:
1 egg white
4-5 drops of Lemon juice
How to:
Mix well to unify. Apply for 15 minutes and rinse.
Note: If you mix the egg yolk with 1 tsp of almond oil, instead of lemon, you have a mask for dry skins. Apply for 15 minutes and rinse well.
Frequency: 1-3 times a week.

WHITENING MASK-2
ALL SKIN TYPES, REDNESS
ANTI-WRINKLE, COLLAGEN REPRODUCTION, FIRMING, RESILI-ENCE, SHINE, SMOOTHING, TIGHTENING, WHITENING
Ingredients:
2 tbsp strawberry pulp
2 tbsp Yogurt

4-5 drops of Lemon juice

How to:

Mash the strawberries. Use quite ripe strawberries, to be mashed easily with a fork. Otherwise, put them in the blender. Mix well all the ingredients until you get a paste. Apply on your face and neck for 20 minutes, and rinse well as usual.

Note: Strawberry is one of the most contaminated with pesticide fruits, so better use organic.

Frequency: 2-3 times a week.

WHITENING MASK-3
ALL SKIN TYPES, DILATED PORES
ANTI-WRINKLE, NOURISH, SHINE, WHITENING

Ingredients:

½ tsp Lemon juice

1 tsp Orange juice

3 ripe Strawberries

¼ ripe Avocado flesh

How to:

Mash the strawberries and the avocado, add the lemon and orange juice and mix well into a fine paste. Apply for 20 minutes and rinse as usual.

Note: A balanced mask that nourishes while it soothes skin redness. Remember to use organic fruits if possible.

Frequency: 1 time per week.

WRINKLE FREE NIGHT-MASK
NORMAL, OILY and COMBINATION SKINS
ANTI-AGING, ANTI-WRINKLE, NOURISHING, SKIN IMPROVEMENT

Ingredients:

1tbsp fresh Milk

A few drops of fresh squeezed Lemon

How to:

Mix and apply. Rinse when it dries or let it stay on your face all night.

Note: Simple, quick and easy, to smooth the wrinkles... away!

Frequency: Repeat every night before you go to bed.

Skin Problems and Needs

Acne: aloe, apple vinegar, brewer's yeast, cabbage, Calendula oil, carrot, chamomile, cinnamon, grapefruit, honey, lettuce, mango, melon, rose water, sandalwood, tomato, turmeric, yogurt
Pages: 20, 21, 22, 25, 30, 35, 36, 37, 41, 45, 47, 49

Anti-aging: almond oil, aloe, apple, banana, brewer's yeast, chamomile, cocoa, cranberry, cucumber, fig, green tea, honey, lemon, milk, oat, olive oil, orange, peach, spinach, sweet potato, tomato
Pages: 20, 23, 24, 25, 26, 27, 28, 29, 30, 31, 32, 33, 37, 38, 39, 40, 41, 43, 45, 46, 48, 50, 51, 52, 54

Antiseptic: apple vinegar, chamomile, cinnamon, grapefruit, green tea, honey, lemon, rose water
Pages: 20, 21, 25, 30, 36, 43, 44, 45, 50

Anti-wrinkle: banana, chamomile, cranberry, kiwi, lemon, mango, milk, pomegranate, sandalwood, spinach, strawberries, sweet potato, watermelon
Pages: 22, 23, 26, 28, 31, 33, 42, 45, 49, 50, 53, 54

Balancing: apple, lettuce, rose water
Pages: 20, 27

Blackheads: baking soda, strawberries
Pages: 46, 53

Broken Blood vessels: lettuce, rose water
Pages: 48

Brown spots: lemon
Pages: 44, 45, 53

Burns: aloe, baking soda, cucumber, grapes, lemon, lettuce, pomegranate, potato, yogurt
Pages: 23, 30, 42, 45, 46, 47, 48, 49, 52

Cell reproduction: aloe, dark chocolate, kiwi, mango, milk, oat, pumpkin seeds, rose water
Pages: 24, 26, 31, 33, 38, 39, 43

Cleansing: aloe, apple, carrot, clay, cranberry, cucumber, fig, honey, kiwi, lemon, lettuce, oat, pomegranate, tomato
Pages: 21, 23, 26, 27, 28, 29, 30, 31, 34, 38, 40, 44, 45, 46, 48, 49, 50, 51, 53

Collagen reproduction: aloe, apple, cocoa, grape, kiwi, melon, strawberries, sweet potato, yogurt
Pages: 23, 34, 37, 38, 42, 49, 50, 53

Colour irregularities: carrot, turmeric, yogurt
Pages: 23, 33, 45, 47

Cracked skin: dark chocolate, sandalwood
Pages: 31, 43

Dark circles: almond oil, chamomile
Pages: 32

Dehydrated skin: almond oil, sandalwood, vegetable glycerin, yogurt
Pages: 32, 43, 47

Delicate skin: green tea, tomato
Pages: 38, 43

Detoxification: clay, dark chocolate, pumpkin seeds
Pages: 20, 39, 43

Dilated pores: orange, strawberries
Pages: 25, 54

Itching: aloe, baking soda, cabbage, Calendula oil, mint, sandalwood
Pages: 35, 37, 46, 51

Moisture: aloe, avocado, banana, Calendula oil, chamomile, cocoa, cranberry, cucumber, dark chocolate, egg, green tea, honey, lettuce, melon, milk, oat, papaya, peach, pumpkin seeds, rose water, sandalwood, strawberries, turmeric, vegetable glycerine, watermelon, yogurt
Pages: 20, 22, 23, 24, 26, 29, 30, 31, 32, 33, 34, 38, 39, 40, 42, 43, 44, 45, 47, 49, 51, 52, 53

Nourishment: apple, avocado, brewer's yeast, clay, cucumber, dark chocolate, egg, honey, milk, mint, oat, olive oil, pumpkin, pumpkin seeds, yogurt
Pages: 20, 21, 22, 23, 24, 25, 26, 27, 28, 29, 30, 31, 32, 33, 36, 37, 39, 40, 41, 43, 47, 52, 53

Oiliness: clay, egg white, kiwi, lemon, lettuce, melon, mint, oat, orange
Pages: 20, 25, 27, 28, 29, 30, 31, 37, 42, 44, 51, 53

Pimples: cinnamon, parsley
Pages: 21, 36

Pollution: honey

Premature aging: mango, cocoa, cranberry
Pages: 23, 45

Psoriasis: lemon, carrot

Puffy eyes: avocado, chamomile, cucumber
Pages: 32

Redness: aloe, brewer's yeast, kiwi, spinach, strawberries, yogurt
Pages: 26, 38, 41, 42, 49, 53

Refreshing: aloe, cucumber, grapefruit, melon, rose water, strawberries, yogurt
Pages: 20, 26, 32, 34, 45, 49

Rejuvenate: cucumber, cranberry, papaya, turmeric, yogurt
Pages: 22, 32, 33, 45, 47

Resilience: aloe, apple vinegar, banana, cucumber, grape, kiwi, melon, olive oil, strawberries, yogurt
Pages: 23, 25, 24, 26, 30, 32, 33, 37, 38, 39, 42, 42, 45, 49, 53

Reconstructing: avocado, Calendula oil, grape, milk, papaya
Pages: 22, 25, 28, 32, 37, 38, 54

Sensitive skin: aloe, chamomile, green tea, spinach, tomato
Pages: 38, 41, 43

Shine: almond oil, banana, clay, cranberry, dark chocolate, egg whites, grape, kiwi, lemon, mango, mint, papaya, pumpkin seeds, rose water, sandalwood, strawberries
Pages: 25, 26, 27, 28, 29, 31, 32, 33, 34, 37, 39, 41, 43, 44, 45, 49, 50, 53, 54

Skin disorders: cabbage, carrot, Calendula oil, chamomile, cinnamon, grape, lemon, mint, pomegranate, sandalwood
Pages: 23, 35, 36, 36, 37, 44

Skin texture improvement: avocado, chamomile, cocoa, dark chocolate, lemon, milk, olive oil, sweet potato, turmeric, watermelon
Pages: 23, 26, 31, 32, 37, 40, 43, 47, 48, 50, 53, 54

Smoothness: aloe, apple, banana, brewer's yeast, Calendula oil, clay, cocoa, cranberry, cucumber, mango, sandalwood, strawberries, vegetable glycerin, yogurt
Pages: 22, 24, 25, 26, 31, 32, 36, 38, 39, 41, 45, 49, 51, 52, 53

Solar protection: green tea, honey, peach, tomato
Pages: 43

Soothing: aloe, apple, mango, mint, olive oil, orange, potato, rose water, yogurt
Pages: 21, 23, 26, 29, 30, 37, 38, 47, 49

Sunburn: aloe, baking soda, cucumber, grape, lemon, lettuce, potato, pomegranate
Pages: 22, 30, 38, 42, 46, 48, 49

Tightening: clay, egg white, papaya, strawberries, watermelon, yogurt
Pages: 26, 27, 28, 33, 34, 42, 43, 51, 53

Tired skin: aloe, egg, milk
Pages: 24, 49, 51

Tonic: clay, cucumber, egg, mint, lemon, milk
Pages: 24, 26, 27, 31, 32, 34, 45, 51, 52, 53

Whitening: lemon, strawberries
Pages: 33, 34, 53, 54

Wrinkles: almond oil, lemon, milk
Pages: 54

All skin types:
Pages: 22, 24, 25, 26, 29, 32, 33, 39, 41, 42, 45, 47, 48, 49, 50, 51, 52, 53, 54

Combination skin:
Pages: 23, 27, 28, 31, 40, 42, 44, 49, 5, 51, 53, 54

Ingredients and Their Properties

Almond oil: My beloved almonds! Almond oil is amazingly beneficial for the skin and the hair.

It contains: Vitamins A, E, B1, B2, B6, minerals such as calcium, chloride, magnesium, phosphorus. Rich in fatty acids.

Benefits: Almond oil provides hydration and shine. Regenerates the skin, soothes irritations and inflammations, tightens skin pores and relieves dryness. It has antioxidant, anti-aging properties and maintains the skin PH to normal. It also helps against the dark circles under the eyes.

Pages: 32, 37, 37, 39, 41, 43, 46

Aloe: An almost magical plant!

It contains: Aloe is a major source of vitamins, such as B, C, E and beta-carotene, and also minerals and trace elements such as magnesium, manganese, zinc, calcium, iron and selenium, and amino acids that build proteins. It is also rich in polysaccharides, sterols, anthraquinones (pain killing substances) and salicylic acid.

Benefits: It cleanses the skin, stimulates cell reproduction, and heals tissues and wounds. Aloe has antimicrobial, antibiotic and antioxidant action. It is ideal for skin irritation, burns and other skin problems such as itching, allergies, bites, even fungal infections etc, because it cools and soothes the skin. Hydrates, softens, increases collagen production, thus slows down the aging process. Finally, it is also used in the treatment of acne.

Pages: 24, 35, 38, 46, 48, 49

Apple: One apple each day and the doctor go away!

It contains: Vitamins A, C, calcium, phosphorus, iron, potassium, folic acid, biotin, malic acid.

Benefits: The malic acid exfoliates gently and makes the skin softer, gives glow to dull skin, while the pectin soothes and strengthens. Apple cleanses in depth and brightens. The

antioxidant properties and the ability to stimulate the production of collagen, define apple as a perfect anti-aging ingredient. It also nourishes, stimulates and balances the skin PH.
Pages: 29, 31, 33, 37

Apple vinegar: Deliscious in salads, but it can also be very beneficial for the health and the skin!

It contains: Minerals such as sodium, potassium, calcium, phosphorus, copper and iron. Ascorbic acid, riboflavin, nicotinic and acetic acid.

Benefits: Apple vinegar is a natural antibacterial and antiseptic, ideal for skin suffering from acne. It helps preserve skin's resilience while it contains enzymes which help the skin to expel the dead cells.
Pages: 21, 25, 30

Avocado: One of the most suitable ingredients for face masks, not only for its nourishing properties but for the buttery texture too.

It contains: 20 Vitamins and minerals such as B1, B2, B3, B5, C, E-biotin, carotenoids, folic acid and potassium. Rich in beta-sitosterol, glutathione, and fibre.

Benefits: It restores the normal texture and colour of dry skin. Anti-aging, with moisturising and healing properties. Good for puffy eyes too. A complete skin nourishment.
Pages: 23, 32, 38, 40, 54

Baking soda: sodium bicarbonate $NaHCO_3$.

Benefits: Relieves itching caused by insect bites, pain from sunburn, while it soothes irritation. Useful in cases of skin dryness. Baking soda has exfoliating properties, removes dirt, dead cells and blackheads.
Pages: 46, 48

Banana: A perfect snack for the skin!

It contains: Vitamins A, B, C and D, riboflavin, niacin, thiamine, iron, copper, zinc, pantothenic acid, phosphorus, calcium, magnesium, potassium and fibre.

Benefits: Banana gives shine and makes the skin soft and resilient. It nourishes, moisturizes and soothes, while it has anti-wrinkle properties.

Pages: 23, 25, 32, 39, 45

Brewer's yeast
It contains: Vitamins D, E, B1, B2, B3, B5, B6, amino acids and minerals.
Benefits: Anti-aging. Nourishes the skin and smoothes wrinkles. It has anti-inflammatory action in juvenile acne and skin eczema.
Pages: 35, 36, 41

Cabbage
It contains: Vitamins A and C, folic acid, phosphorus, sulphur, iodine, potassium, sodium, magnesium and manganese.
Benefits: Effective in the treatment of skin rashes such as eczema, psoriasis, acne and insect bites.
Pages: 35, 37

Calendula Oil: As if you had baby's skin!
It contains: Saponins, flavonoids, vitamin C, calcium, carotenes and significant amounts of silicon.
Benefits: It helps against skin irritation, bites and wounds, eczema, acne and infections. It is good for all skin types and especially beneficial for skin dryness. Calendula oil has anti-inflammatory and healing properties. Beneficial for all skin issues because it has the ability to regenerate the tissues. Hydrates the skin and makes it supple.
Pages: 36, 46

Carrot: Makes your skin beautiful!
It contains: Carrot has a sufficient amount of vitamins B1, B2, K, C, E and niacin. It is the richest vegetable source of beta - carotene (provitamin A) and an excellent source of antioxidants. Carrots also contain manganese, potassium, calcium,

magnesium, phosphorus, sodium, iron, zinc, copper and selenium.

Benefits: Carrots clean the skin, helps against acne and colour irregularities. Suitable for dry skin. It also helps in cases of psoriasis.

Pages: 23, 35

Chamomile: The humble herb with the noble properties!

It contains: Vitamins C, B1, tannins, salicylic acid, coumarin derivatives (vitamin K antagonists), copper, potassium, zinc, iron, phosphorus, magnesium,. It is also rich in antioxidants called flavones and glycosides (powerful antioxidants of the flavonoids family)

Benefits: It helps against several skin problems, such as acne or infections by fungi, while it relieves the irritated skin. Chamomile improves dark circles and eye puffiness. Ideal for sensitive skin types. It has antioxidant, antiseptic and anti-irritant properties. Phytosterols contained, have a direct anti-wrinkle and moisturizing effect, and improve the skin tone.

Pages: 44

Cinnamon: Spicy and healing!

It contains: Vitamin A, niacin, pantothenic acid and pyridoxine and volatile oils. Excellent source of manganese, iron, calcium, fibre. Cinnamon also contains flavonoid phenolics and antioxidants such as carotenoids.

Benefits: Acne, pimples, eczema, lichens and skin infections. Antiseptic.

Pages: 21, 36

Clay: There are many types of clays with different properties. However, some of the major clay benefits are the following:

Benefits: Proper for oily and combination skins, or acne problems. Cleanses, tones, softens and nourishes the skin. It absorbs oiliness (montmorillonite: green clay of Provence) and helps the skin to expel toxins, sebum and dirt (Illite: Green Clay). It also helps the skin to heal (kaolinite: white clay)

Cocoa: Tasty and nourishing!
It contains: B complex vitamins. Rich in flavonoids with antioxidant activity. It also contains phosphorus, potassium, magnesium and fibre.
Benefits: Slows down skin aging, maintains the levels of skin collagen, moisturises and improves skin's texture.

Cranberry: Small but powerful!
It contains: Vitamins C, D, iron, potassium, flavonoids.
Benefits: Antioxidant. Removes dead skin cells, hydrates and reduces wrinkles. For shiny, smooth and healthy skin.

Cucumber: The ultimate refreshing!
It contains: Vitamins C, B1, B2, B3, B5, fibre, folic acid, calcium, protein, fat, carbohydrates, iron, phosphorus, potassium, sugars, magnesium, zinc, manganese and silicon.
Benefits: Cleans and revitalizes the skin, stimulates the eyes and reduces puffiness due to ascorbic and caffeic acids, while it relieves burns and irritation. Moisturizes, helps exfoliation and it is an excellent nutrient for the skin, leaving it soft and tender. The cucumber juice has tonic, antioxidant, emollient and moisturizing properties.

Dark Chocolate: Sweet and smooth!
It contains: The dark chocolate contains cocoa, cocoa butter and a little sugar. Magnesium, caffeine, theobromine, Phenylethylamine.
Benefits: It has antioxidant, anti-aging properties. Dark chocolate nourishes and moisturizes dry and cracked skin. Stimulates the growth of skin cells and improves the skin texture. Detoxifies and brightens.

Egg: Nourishes all types of skin.

It contains: Vitamins A, D, E, B complex, including folic acid. Potassium, iron, phosphorus, iodine and zinc.

Benefits: The egg proteins are quite beneficial for the skin. It stimulates the cell renewal process. The egg white tones, tightens and has bleaching properties, while the yolk, rich in vitamin A, nourishes and moisturizes.

Pages: 22, 23, 24, 27, 28, 29, 33, 34, 37, 40, 42, 44, 51, 53

Fig: A sweet summer friend!

It contains: Vitamins A, C and B1, B2, iron, magnesium, potassium, calcium, phosphorus, manganese, sodium,. Figs are a rich source of fibre.

Benefits: Anti-aging action. The tiny seeds exfoliate and cleanse the skin gently while they remove dead cells.

Pages: 40, 46

Grape: A fruit of the Gods!

It contains: Rich in vitamins A, C, B, calcium, iron, phosphorus, potassium and polyphenols.

Beneficial: Skin diseases, diseases of the eyes, local pain, even burns. Protects the collagen and elastin of the tissues, and provides firming and shine.

Pages: 22, 49

Grapefruit: A natural tonic for skin and hair.

It contains: Vitamins A, B, C and minerals such as calcium, manganese, iron, magnesium, potassium and phosphorus.

Benefits: It has antimicrobial, antiseptic and disinfectant properties. Grapefruit is refreshing and invigorating. It is also said that grapefruit extract and seeds can fight all sorts of eczema.

Pages: 20, 25

Green Tea: The antioxidant ally!

It contains: Antioxidants such as polyphenols, tannins, flavonols, other flavonoids, perfume oils, saponins, amino acids and also metals (iron, copper, zinc, potassium, phosphorus, fluorine), vitamins (K, A, B, E, C), etc.

Benefits: Anti-aging, antioxidant, antiseptic, tonic, improves blood circulation. Ideal for sensitive or irritated skin, with moisturizing properties. Protects against solar radiation.

Pages: 43, 50

Honey: Sweet nutrition for your skin!

It contains: Multitude of vitamins, such as vitamin B6, thiamin, niacin, riboflavin, pantothenic acid. Minerals such as calcium, copper, iron, magnesium, manganese, phosphorus, zinc, sodium and potassium. Water, amino and organic acids.

Benefits: It has antibacterial effects, fights free radicals, protects against solar radiation and pollution. Moisturizes, ideal for dry skin. Fights infections and rashes, while it cleans the skin deeply. Honey has healing and nourishing properties. Its antibacterial activity helps against acne.

Pages: 21, 22, 23, 26, 27, 28, 29, 30, 31, 33, 34, 35, 36, 38, 40, 41, 44, 45, 47, 48, 49, 50, 51, 52

Kiwi: Sweet & sour! Miraculous!

It contains: Vitamins C, E, K, potassium, organic acids, omega-3, choline, potassium, phosphorus, iron, calcium, magnesium, copper, zinc.

Benefits: Makes the skin radiant and durable. Kiwi activates cell and collagen production, therefore it reduces wrinkles. It cleans, exfoliates gently and makes the skin elastic. Soothes redness, brightens and removes the oiliness gloss.

Pages: 42

Lemon: A fruit with countless applications and benefits!

It contains: Vitamins B, C, 22 anti-cancer compounds such as limonene. Riboflavin, minerals such as calcium, phosphorus, magnesium, as well as proteins and carbohydrates.

Benefits: Vitamin C fights against aging and helps with wrinkles and spot removal. Very beneficial to sunburns, bunions, psoriasis, and even freckles. Cleans and whitens the skin.

A natural antiseptic for treating skin disorders. Brightens and tones the skin quality.

Pages: 20, 25, 28, 29, 33, 34, 35, 36, 37, 41, 44, 45, 48, 51, 52, 53, 54

Lettuce: Not just for salads!

It contains: Vitamins A, B, C, D and E, Calcium, Phosphorus, Potassium, Cobalt, Copper, Chlorine, Iodine, Iron, Zinc, Magnesium, Manganese.

Benefits: Soothes the burns. Helps in cases of acne and excess oil. Removes sebum and dead cells. Also helps against spider veins. Antioxidant action. Absorbs excess oil and balances the skin PH.

Pages: 48

Milk: Always prefer organic milk.

Pages: 23, 25, 26, 27, 31, 33, 37, 40, 54

Almond milk: Vitamins A, E, B2 or riboflavin. A rich source of calcium, magnesium, manganese, copper, tryptophan, phosphorus. An antioxidant that protects both cells and tissues. It repairs free radicals and keeps the skin healthy, clean, bright and youthful. Moisturizes.

Goat milk: Vitamins A, B1, B2, C, D, calcium, iron, magnesium, potassium, sodium, phosphorus. Goat milk provides softness and elasticity to the skin. Moisturizes, protects and strengthens the skin and the cells. Nourishes, regenerates, tones and pampers the tired and dull skin.

Donkey milk: Contains 60 times more vitamin C than cow's milk, vitamins A, B1, B2, B6, D, and E and rich in calcium, magnesium, phosphorus, sodium, zinc and iron. Helps firming and skin cell regeneration. Increases the tissues that support the skin, makes it smoother, tight, stretchy, velvety with youthful radiance. It has emollient and regenerating properties.

Mango: An exotic and nutritious fruit!

It contains: Vitamins A, C, B complex. A rich source of beta carotene and lycopene, calcium and magnesium.

Benefits: Relieves clogged pores and acne, while it makes the skin radiant and soft. Promotes cell regeneration and slows the premature aging
Pages: 22

Melon: The golden summer treasure!
It contains: Vitamins A, B1, B2, B3, C, beta carotene, high potassium content, thiamine, niacin.
Benefits: Contributes to collagen synthesis, stimulates the skin and reduces acne. Refreshing, moisturizing and emollient, helps to combat oiliness.
Pages: 34

Mint: One of the most famous herbs!
It contains: Vitamins A and C and Vitamin B2 in smaller quantities, manganese, iron, potassium and calcium.
Benefits: Soothes itching, pain and irritated skin caused from various skin diseases. Nourishes dull skin and gives shine, while it reduces oiliness. Tones the skin.
Pages: 26, 47, 51

Oats: Serve your skin a nice... breakfast!
It contains: Rich in vitamins B, E, K, biotin, folic acid, fibre. Minerals such as calcium, copper, iron, magnesium, manganese, phosphorus, potassium, selenium, silicon, zinc. Saponins, amino acids
Benefits: Nourishes and helps cell reproduction. The saponins absorb skin oils, while the antioxidant elements empower the oats with an anti-aging action. Hydrates and exfoliates.
Pages: 26, 29, 30, 31, 33, 51, 53

Olive oil: The green gold!
It contains: Rich in antioxidants, such as vitamin E and polyphenols, and chlorophyll. Moreover, it contains vitamin C and minerals like sodium, potassium and iron.
Benefits: Protects against dryness and improves the skin texture because of its soothing properties. It has anti-aging ef-

fects, thanks to the antioxidants it contains. Olive oil soothes the skin, nourishes and provides elasticity.
Pages: 23, 30, 37, 39, 40, 42, 46, 48, 49

Orange: Drink an orange juice every day!
It contains: Vitamins A, B1, C. Orange is a good source of amino acids, beta-carotene, folic acid, pectin, potassium, calcium, iron, iodine, phosphorus, manganese, sodium, chlorine, and zinc.
Benefits: Orange is an antioxidant fruit. It has soothing and astringent properties that help to strengthen the oily skin and dilated pores.
Pages: 25, 29, 36, 54

Papaya: It will make you shine!
It contains: Vitamins C, A, E, many nutrients and antioxidants. Rich in beta-carotene, flavonoids, minerals, potassium, magnesium and fibre.
Benefits: Prevents, heals and restores. Exfoliates lightly the skin. Gives a natural face-lifting, rejuvenation, hydration, radiance and freshness.
Pages: 34

Parsley: In ancient Greece, parsley was used by Hippocrates, exclusively, as a medicinal plant.
It contains: Parsley is rich in minerals and vitamins. It contains more iron than any other green vegetable, and also great amounts of vitamins A and B and three times more vitamin C than citrus fruits.
Benefits: Parsley oil has vasodilating and healing action. Eliminates pimples.
Pages: 21, 37

Peach: For velvet skin!
It contains: fibre, protein, vitamins E, C, biotin, sugar, iron, potassium, phosphorus and calcium.
Benefits: It has moisturizing and anti-aging properties. It also protects against solar radiation.

Pages: 44, 48, 50

Pomegranate: Forever young!
It contains: Rich in vitamins A, C, E, folic acid, iron, potassium and fibre, tannins, anthocyanins, ellagic acid.
Benefits: Antimicrobial, anti-inflammatory, astringent and healing properties. Cleans and protects the skin. Helps with burns and herpes virus treatment. Reduces wrinkles, ulcers and skin blemishes.
Pages: 23, 28, 30

Potato: Soothes and relieves.
It contains: Vitamins C, B1, B6 and folic acid, niacin, thiamine, riboflavin. A good source of potassium.
Benefits: Relieves immediately the pain and irritation of burns. The potato starch soothes the inflamed tissues by its emollient and analgesic action. Helps in the cases of face lichen; the red, dry and rough spots on the cheeks, chin and nose.
Pages: 37

Pumpkin: Making a pie? Save some pumpkin for your face mask!
It contains: Rich in beta-carotene. Excellent source of vitamins B1, B3, B5, B6, C. Rich in magnesium, potassium and fibre. It also contains copper, omega-3 fatty acids, starch.
Benefits: Exfoliates and nourishes the skin with vitamins and enzymes. Ideal for dry and dull skin.
Pages: 33, 46

Pumpkin seeds: The natural... Botox!
It contains: Their oil is rich in unsaturated fatty acids and iron. They also contain zinc, copper, magnesium, manganese and phosphorus, selenium, vitamins A, E, C, K, some of the vitamin B complex and folic acid.
Benefits: The pumpkin seeds are very nutritious for the skin, they keep it vigorous and help the rapid cell regenera-

tion. Fatty acids assist in skin moisturizing, but also in the elimination of toxins.
Pages: 39

Rose water: A fountain of freshness!
Benefits: Brightens the skin. Rose water has antiseptic properties. Stimulates and refreshes while it soothes and moisturizes. It also helps the quick healing of acne scars and marks. Rose water stimulates blood circulation and eliminates the signs of broken blood vessels. It balances the skin pH and enhances the process of cell regeneration.
Pages: 35, 38, 41

Sandalwood: A valuable essential oil!
Benefits: It keeps the skin soft and hydrated. Beneficial for skin disorders such as acne and eczema, because it relieves itching and inflammation. Its moisturizing properties help the dry or cracked skin, scars, wrinkles and give shine.
Pages: 22, 36

Spinach: Don't forget to eat your spinach!
It contains: Vitamins A, B, C, K, fibre, iron, manganese, calcium, folic acid, carotene and lutein.
Benefits: Antioxidant. Strengthens the skin defence, reduces sensitivity and redness.
Pages: 26, 41

Strawberries: Defeat the signs of aging!
It contains: Vitamin C, K, B5, B6, potassium, manganese, riboflavin, folic acid, magnesium, copper and antioxidants.
Benefits: Due to the high content of vitamin C, strawberries reduce wrinkles and improve skin dryness. Moisturize and soften the skin. They remove dead cells and blackheads without drying the skin. A natural exfoliant that cleans and refreshes the skin, reduces redness, tightens the pores, lightens and brightens the face. Activates the production of collagen and elastin.

Pages: 26, 53,53

Sweet Potato: Miraculous for health and beauty!
It contains: Vitamins A, B, C, K, omega-3 fatty acids, magnesium, phosphorus, potassium, sodium and zinc. High carotenoid content.
Benefits: It helps wound healing and collagen production. Anti-aging. Smoothes wrinkles and makes the skin look younger.
Pages: 50

Tomato: Wonderful, red tomatoes! They can do skin miracles!
It contains: Vitamin A and C, microelements, lycopene, beta-carotene, metals such as iron, potassium, magnesium, calcium, phosphorus.
Benefits: It is a powerful antioxidant, therefore, a perfect anti-aging cosmetic ingredient. Beta-carotene and lycopene are enhancing the melanin production, and they function as a photoprotector. The tomato has cleansing and abrasive action, and it is ideal for delicate, dull skin and acne problems.
Pages: 20, 38, 43, 45

Turmeric: A health secret!
It contains: The active ingredient in turmeric is the curcumin substance.
Benefits: Helps the healing of skin wounds, while it treats the scars from acne and skin discoloration. Improves skin's appearance and texture. Pampers, rejuvenates and moisturizes.
Pages: 21, 47, 52

Vegetable Glycerin: Pure for homemade cosmetics.
Benefits: Softens, moisturizes and keeps skin soft and hydrated. Ideal for dry and dehydrated skin. Better use it mixed with other ingredients.
Pages: 51

Watermelon: A hydrating treasure!

It contains: Water, lycopene, Vitamins A, C and B6, beta-carotene, thiamine and potassium.

Benefits: The high water content hydrates the skin and gives a youthful appearance. Tightens the pores, reduces the wrinkles and improves skin's texture.

Pages: 42

Yogurt: For masks with great texture.

It contains: Calcium, phosphorus, potassium and vitamins A and B.

Benefits: Nourishes and moisturizes the dehydrated skin. Regenerates and rejuvenates and makes the skin smoother. Yogurt's refreshing texture, soothes skin irritation and redness. It also has a firming action due to the lactic acid it contains, while it helps against acne because of the probiotic antibacterial action.

Pages: 20, 22, 23, 26, 29, 30, 32, 33, 38, 42, 45, 47, 48, 49, 52, 53

Disclaimer

The above information is a sharing of traditional knowledge and experiences for educational and informational purposes. It does not constitute medical diagnosis or medication recommendation. This book is not intended to substitute professional diagnosis and treatment. Also, is not intended to replace any medication you are already taking or the advice of your doctor.

The author and the publishers disclaim any warranties and are not liable for excessive and careless use, for any incidental or consequential damage connected direct or indirectly with the content of this ebook, or the ignoring of the recommendations of your doctor.

The liability, use, misuse, negligence of any recipe, instruction or ideas given in this book is under the total responsibility of the reader.

Author and publisher disclaim also any warranties for the accuracy of the external links content.

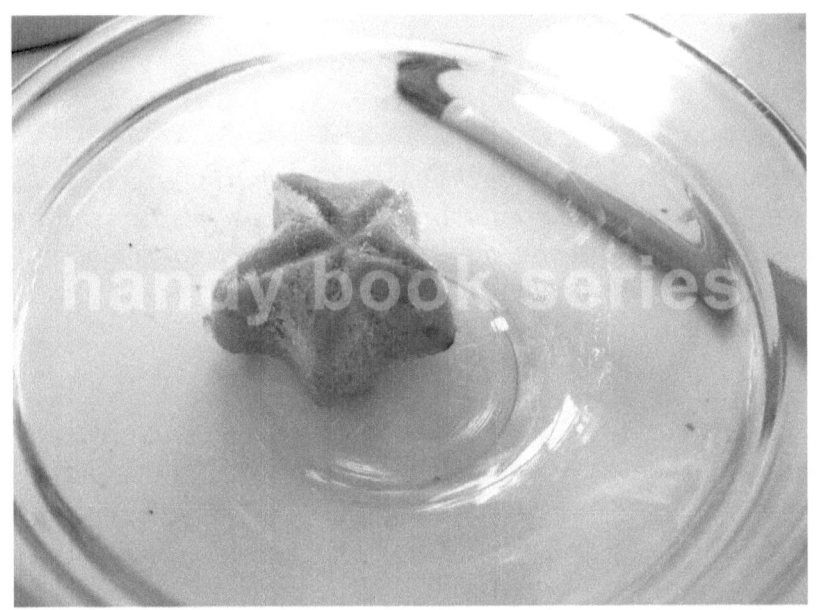

Visit : http://evelinbooks.wordpress.com

*for updates, new beauty and cooking recipes,
tips and instructions for homemade products,
ideas sharing and lots of colourful images!*

"I bought this book for my girlfriend who is studying as a beautician and she found the 80 recipes in this book very useful. I'm no beautician and I found it amazing there are so many natural combinations available. Good practical read. "
[JF. Review from 1st digital edition]

"This is an amazing book. Who knew there were so many ways to do a mask: she includes a sunburn mask, a spider veins mask and an acne mask. There are also face-lifting, forever-young and other youth restoring masks.

This book is well researched, well written and with 80 to choose from, there are masks for everyone. "
[Daniel Speraw, author. Review from 1st digital edition]

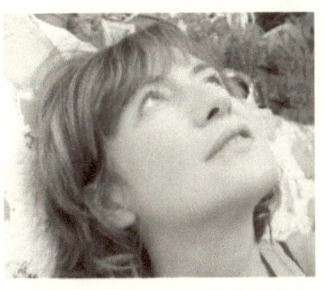

Hello!
The major advantage of making homemade cosmetics, is that you have total control of the ingredients you use. Products such as masks, creams and lotions, provide nutrition to the skin, so they have to be pure, organic and free of toxins.
I hope that my new book, "80 recipes for beauty face masks", has already stimulated your appetite for healthy, natural and... tasty cosmetics!
Spend some quality time to treat yourself, in a world of wonderful smells, bright colours and delightful flavours!

80 Recipes for Beauty Face Masks

www.ingramcontent.com/pod-product-compliance
Lightning Source LLC
Chambersburg PA
CBHW020348290526
45785CB00005B/2187